Why Live
How Suicide
Becomes
an Epidemic

I0110003

Helen C. Epstein

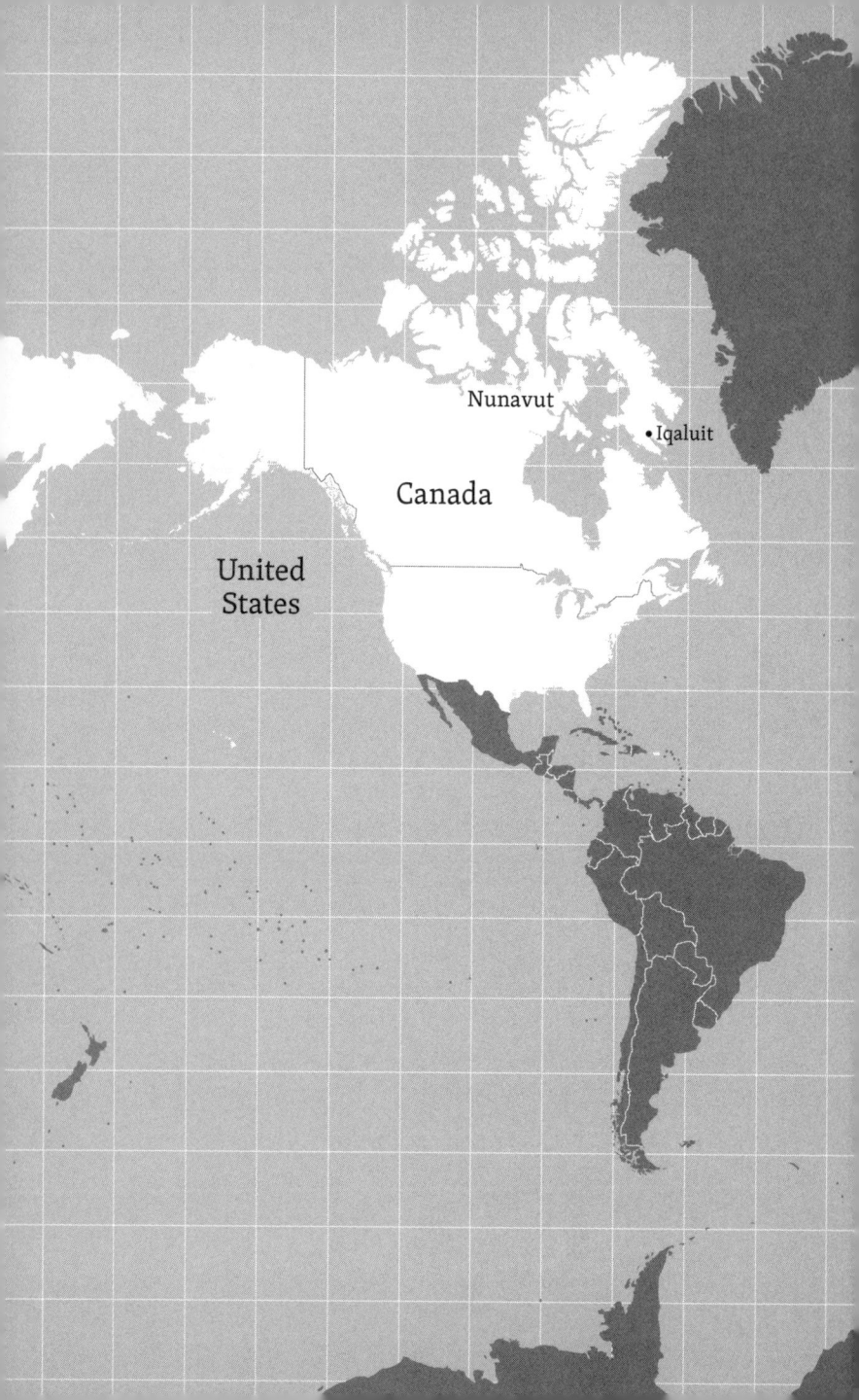

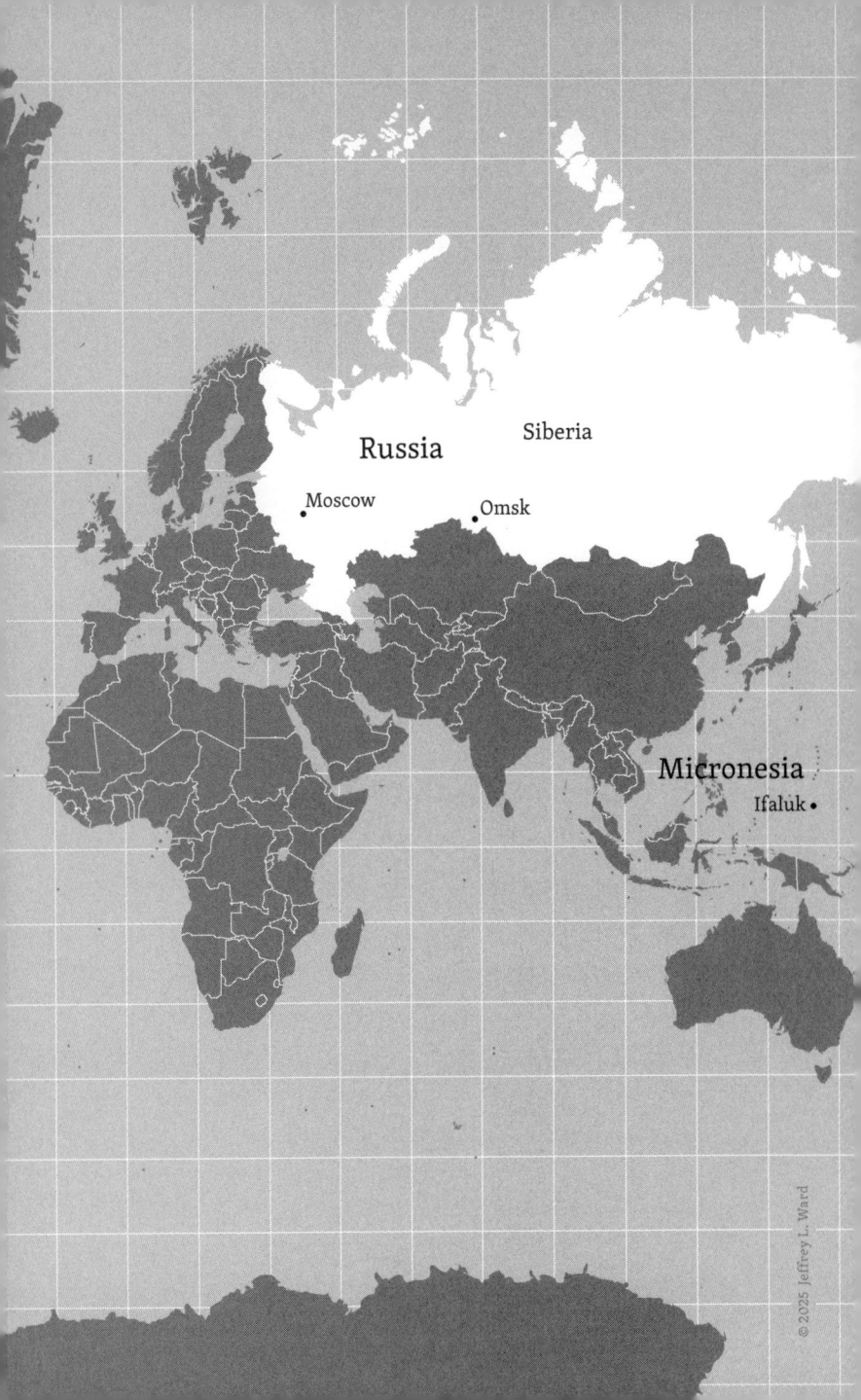

Russia

Siberia

Moscow

Omsk

Micronesia

Ifaluk

© 2025 Jeffrey L. Ward

Why Live
How Suicide Becomes an Epidemic
Copyright © 2025 by Helen C. Epstein
All rights reserved

Published by Columbia Global Reports
91 Claremont Avenue, Suite 515
New York, NY 10027
globalreports.columbia.edu

Library of Congress Cataloging-in-Publication Data Available Upon Request

ISBN 979-8-987053-74-4 (paperback)

Book design by Kelly Winton
Map design by Jeffrey L. Ward
Author photograph by Petr Petr

Printed in the United States of America

To Robert Silvers, in memory.

CONTENTS

Introduction

I'd known the writer Jean Stein since I was six. She and my mother had been friends. She had talent, beauty, money, and children and grandchildren who loved her. Her suicide stunned me.

I'd known she was depressed. About a year before she died, we were having dinner with another friend when Jean suddenly fell silent. I tried helplessly to fill the conversation, and she struggled to smile, but something was clearly wrong.

"What is it? Are you okay?" I asked after our friend had gone home.

She shook her head and looked down at her own clasped hands. Then her lips parted, as if she were about to speak, but no words came out.

I wish I'd understood then how confusing suicidal feelings are, and how hard to describe. Those who experience them often don't understand what's going on themselves. "Black choler," as the seventeenth-century British author Robert Burton described it in his famous tome, *The Anatomy of Melancholy*. Psychologist and suicide expert Edwin Shneidman called it "psychache," an excruciating feeling of utter loss, like being trapped in a "whirlpool of [emotional] confusion," unable to think about anything except one's own misery, from which death seems the only escape.

Like many people whose friends or relatives have taken their own lives, I can't stop wondering whether there was something I could have said or done that might have made a difference. There is no way to predict who will die by suicide. Millions of Americans suffer from severe depression, but only about one in a thousand of them take their own lives in any given year. "Only in retrospect," the Israeli psychologist Yossi Levi-Belz told me, "can we look back and wonder if we missed a crucial signal."

This isn't primarily a book about how to prevent suicide. Such a book would have detailed sections about psychotherapy, restrictions on firearms, safety barriers for bridges, and other measures that really do save lives. This book begins upstream, with volition. My aim is to explore why some people want to take their own lives in the first place and how that desire might be reduced, in both individuals and communities. I also hope to give at least partial answers to those who survive.

Since Jean died, I've come to see how suicide often stems from an acute awareness of the self, and the precipitous, sometimes terrifying sense that we are alone in a fragmented, often heartless and pointless-seeming world. I'm far from the first to have made this point. Existentialists and other philosophers— Jean-Paul Sartre, Albert Camus, Friedrich Nietzsche, and Søren Kierkegaard, for example—all grappled with suicide, the self, and modernity. Why live, they asked, now that the mystery of religion had been revealed to be a sham and the world

10   had been stripped of meaning and spirituality by war, indus-
trialization, and other modern ills? They all came to different conclusions, but they boil down to this: have faith anyway
(Kierkegaard); embrace voluntary death if you want to, because
it's the ultimate act of freedom (Nietzsche); find pleasure in the
little things in life, including love, art, and even suffering itself
(Camus); and just do something and don't worry about what
it all means, because, as Camus also maintained, life is absurd
anyway (Sartre).

    Having spent the past few years reading about suicide,
speaking with scores of people who've experienced suicidal
feelings, and having experienced them myself from time to
time, I've come to wonder if the above philosophers, brilliant as
they were, knew what they were talking about—at least when it
comes to this subject. As I've come to understand it, what suicidal people feel is the indifference, not of the universe, but of
those closest to them. They sense that their own feelings don't
matter to the people they care most about. It's the opposite of
what Roquentin, the wandering, blocked writer in Sartre's exis-
tentialist novel *Nausea*, says about it. In the story, he decides
to keep living because no one would care if he died, and his
suicide would therefore be a meaningless gesture. By contrast, studies show that the main reason suicidal people want
to die is precisely because they think no one cares about them.
The indifference of others is a reason to die, not—as Sartre's
Roquentin maintains—to endure. Some suicides even seem
to believe they're doing everyone a favor by taking their own
lives. Psychologist Thomas Joiner, who's been studying suicide for thirty years, calls it a force of nature that distorts people's minds so they become convinced that they are a burden

to others and no one wants them around. In study after study, the most common trigger for suicide is a perceived rupture in a close relationship, either with a lover, parent, or other close relative, that seems irreparable to the suicidal person.

This must sound, well, crazy—especially to those who have lost people to suicide. When someone takes his own life, the grief of parents, lovers, children, and friends can be unspeakable. It's hard to think of anything worse. At a memorial for one young suicide I attended a few years ago, the father of the deceased could barely walk to the altar to light a candle. Everyone was crying.

How could this talented, beautiful young person not know she'd be terribly, horribly missed? That is what I've been trying to get my head around. Most experts attribute suicide to severe mental illness caused by a brain injury or genetic predisposition, or due to some other, as yet unknown, physical or chemical trigger. Severe depression, bipolar disorder, and schizophrenia are all inordinately common among people who die by suicide. Sometimes, the medicines used to treat these illnesses backfire, bringing on suicidal feelings in people who were merely depressed before. Selective serotonin reuptake inhibitors like Prozac, for example, have helped many people, but they have also been shown to double or even triple suicidal attempts that lead to hospital visits and/or death, in depressed teens and young adults.

Severe mental illnesses are no doubt responsible for many, if not most, of the eight hundred thousand or so suicides that occur around the world each year, including, perhaps, those of Jean and that young person whose memorial I attended. But this book is not, primarily, about such cases. Instead, it deals

12   with instances in which the suicide rate of a particular group
jumps—sometimes increasing three- or four-fold or more—in
a short time, meaning it behaves like an epidemic, like malaria
during the rainy season or flu in the fall. Suicide epidemics
unfold more slowly than these microbial plagues—over years or
decades, not weeks or months—but they happen far too quickly
to result from genetic changes, and affect far too many people to
be explained away as spontaneous cases of biologically caused
mental illness or brain injury. The causes therefore must have
something to do with the changing social environment in which
these people live.*

Suicide epidemics have occurred on virtually every conti-
nent. Between the 1820s and World War I, suicides nearly tripled in Belgium, Italy, and France, and quadrupled in Austria.
In the UK, male prisoners are roughly six times, and female
prisoners twenty-four times, more likely to take their own
lives than non-prisoners are, and their risk remains high even
after they are released. In 2014, young veterans of the Iraq and
Afghan wars were roughly five times as likely as same-aged
civilians to take their own lives. The suicide rate doubled among
middle-aged Russians after the collapse of Soviet communism in the early 1990s, and quadrupled in white middle-aged

---

*This book does not deal with copycat behavior. Suicide epidemics are
different from suicide contagion—which refers to suicidal behavior in
the wake of the suicide of friends and acquaintances. According to recent
studies, such contagion is usually limited to suicidal ideation (thinking
about suicide) and attempts, not actual suicides. See, for example, India
Bohanna, "Suicide 'Contagion': What We Know and What We Need to Find
Out," *Canadian Medical Association Journal* 185, no. 10 (2013): 861–862.
https://pmc.ncbi.nlm.nih.gov/articles/PMC3707988/. Suicide clusters—
small numbers of suicides in particular communities—though tragic, are
statistically modest compared to the epidemics discussed here.

working-class Americans after deindustrialization commenced
in the 1970s. Between 1980 and 2003, suicide among Inuit
youths in the Canadian Arctic soared from almost zero to a
rate ten times higher than that of the white majority Canadian
population; similar spikes commenced during the 1970s in
young people living on the Pacific Islands collectively known
as Micronesia; during the 1980s among the Traveller people of England and Ireland; during the 1970s among farmers in
India, Latin America, and the US;* and during the 2000s among
the Acholi people of Uganda and, more recently, among young
Americans, especially Blacks.†

What's scary about this is that it means suicide could come
for any of us. The very existence of suicide epidemics proves
that people with suicidal feelings aren't a species apart. Anyone
can feel suicidal under certain conditions. The aim of this book
is to explore what those conditions are and what has helped
those who survived them endure.

I teach and write about public health and have long been
fascinated by epidemics because they always tell a story. In
most literary depictions of epidemics, such as Albert Camus's
The Plague or Daniel Defoe's *A Journal of the Plague Year*, they
seem to strike from nowhere, but this isn't how epidemics

---

* **In India:** Nanda Kishore Kannuri and Sushrut Jadhav, "Cultivating Distress:
Cotton, Caste and Farmer Suicides in India," *Anthropology & Medicine* 28,
no. 4 (2021): 558–575; **Latin America:** Charlotte Shaw, Jaimee Stuart, Troy
Thomas, and Kairi Kõlves, "Suicidal Behaviour and Ideation in Guyana: A
Systematic Literature Review," *Lancet Regional Health-Americas* 11 (2022):
100253; **and the US:** Debbie Weingarten, "Why Are America's Farmers
Killing Themselves?" *The Guardian*, December 11, 2018.

† Christina Caron, "Why Are More Black Kids Suicidal? A Search for
Answers," *New York Times*, November 18, 2021.

14   typically behave. Individual cases of disease are hard to pre-
      dict. Some of us will become ill tomorrow, but there's no telling
      who. Even those who take risks may well escape the conse-
      quences. Some years back, a British tabloid featured on its
      cover a chain-smoker named Winnie lighting a cigarette with a
      candle on her hundredth birthday cake. But epidemics—which
      affect large numbers of people at certain times and places—
      always happen for a reason. The mass production of cigarettes
      in the early twentieth century, along with their marketing as
      symbols of masculine mystique and women's empowerment,
      helped spark America's lung cancer epidemic; flu cases soar
      around the winter holidays, when people gather indoors for rit-
      ual feasts and celebrations.

      What might cause a suicide epidemic? First, it's import-
      ant to understand what doesn't. Suicide isn't more common
      during wars or where people are poorer or have recently experi-
      enced some environmental disaster like a flood, earthquake, or
      wildfire. Suicide was common among African slaves, especially
      on the ships en route to America and when they first arrived,
      but despite segregation, police brutality, mass incarceration,
      and other outrages, the suicide rate of African Americans has
      been generally lower than that of US whites since recordkeeping
      began in the 1930s. Jews in Nazi-occupied Europe killed them-
      selves in large numbers, inside and outside the concentration
      camps. But their children are no more likely to die by suicide
      than the children of Jews who lived outside Nazi-occupied lands
      at the time.

      What seems to matter is whether people believe some-
      one, somewhere, really cares about and understands them. The
      mental pain that drives suicide is really the flip side of love, says

Israeli neuroscientist Yoram Yovell. "It probably evolved along with motherhood. . . . Inherent in us are very strong emotional forces that function to keep mothers and babies together. When they get too far from each other, they feel mental pain," which we experience when we search for love. This is why "so many children's stories are about a boy looking for his lost mother."

Evidence supports Yovell's theory. A 1999 study found that some 78 percent of high lethality suicide attempters had recently experienced the loss of a close personal relationship, and suicide notes often express love for those left behind. In 2012, Zimri Yaseen and colleagues reported that suicidal people interviewed in emergency rooms were especially likely to report that in the three preceding days, they'd felt "unusually intense or deep feelings of love," which they presumably also felt were not reciprocated.

A great many political suicides—altruists, martyrs, terrorists—also seem to experience such feelings. In childhood, 9/11 hijacker Mohammed Atta, for example, was isolated from other children deliberately by his overbearing father; as a graduate student in Germany, he was taunted by his roommates, and seems to have been an outcast even among his fellow terrorists. Those who knew him say he virtually never laughed, never played games or went dancing, and went to the movies only once and then vowed never to go again. In the years before 9/11, he'd misled his parents into believing he was earning a PhD, even though he was still marooned in a master's program, and seems to have feared the shame and disgrace that would follow if they were to discover the truth.

But why would large groups of people—from the islands of Micronesia to the Arctic Circle, from the cities of post-

16   communist Russia to the towns of contemporary America—
        suddenly begin questioning their most intimate attachments?
        How does love suddenly disappear—or seem to—from the lives
        of thousands of people?

        The hypothesis of this book is that it has to do with how
        we internalize socioeconomic change. The first well-researched
        suicide epidemic occurred across Western Europe during the
        nineteenth century. Intellectuals debated the causes as we
        debate the vicissitudes of the stock market. Rising suicide rates
        were attributed to socialism, atmospheric moisture, the vice of
        masturbation, and the Romantic era inclination to preserve—
        through death—the passions of youth against the onslaught of
        Bourgeois boredom brought on by industrialization and urban
        life. Doctors even searched, in vain, for a suicidogenic organ in
        the cadavers of people who'd died by suicide. But others blamed
        society, that collective property of human groups that shapes
        our thinking and behavior.

        As a Jew growing up in France amid increasing anti-
        Semitism, Émile Durkheim had seen how shared values and
        beliefs buffered his people against the effects of discrimination
        and how anti-Semitism tightened bonds among them. He went
        on to become one of the founders of sociology, which is the study
        of those bonds: what holds us together, what drives us apart, and
        what happens as a result. In his 1897 book, *Suicide*, Durkheim
        theorized that Europe's soaring suicide rate was a manifestation
        of a general process of moral decline signified by waning reli-
        gious faith, the spread of pornography, increases in alcoholism
        and crime, and a rash of anarchist bombings and assassinations
        that threatened to tear Europe apart. He likened it to entropy—
        the universal tendency toward chaos and disorder at the atomic

level discovered by physicists earlier in the century. Appearing
on the eve of humanity's, as yet, bloodiest century, Durkheim's
book seemed to foreshadow the trouble to come.

Durkheim's crucial insight was that suicides increase
wherever society is fragmenting and people are growing more
detached from one another: where divorce rates are higher, for
example, and where Protestants, with their individualistic culture and aloofness from collective ritual, outnumber Catholics.

What is it about fragmenting societies that causes mental pain? Durkheim was vague, even a little loopy, when it came
to explaining this. At the time, psychologists were just dis-
covering the unconscious, which they explored through studies of hypnosis and hallucinations. Durkheim followed this
research closely, and believed that values and meanings flowed
through populations like electrical currents, as if societies had
what scholars Laurent Mucchielli and Marc Renneville refer
to as a "collective soul" that could change people's behavior
through unconscious mechanisms, just as changes in temperature and pressure change the behavior of molecules. Many
late-nineteenth-century scientists believed that our brains
generated signals analogous to radio waves. Alexander Graham
Bell, Nikolai Tesla, and James Clerk Maxwell even wired up
helmets and other gizmos to try to measure them. Mark Twain
told *Harper's Monthly* that thoughts could shoot from brain to
brain, without their owners having to open their mouths to
communicate. Likewise, Durkheim maintained that whatever
suicidal people said about their feelings were just expressions
of resolutions planted in their minds by the vibes of a disintegrating society.

18   The brain-wave theory eventually fell out of fashion. In the 1930s, one of Durkheim's protégés came closer to explaining the psychological effects of social fragmentation. Maurice Halbwachs taught at the University of Strasbourg from 1919 until his death in a Nazi concentration camp in 1945. In 1930, he delivered a series of lectures on suicide at the University of Chicago. He was an uncharismatic teacher, and by the end of the semester, only three students remained. But he was a clearer writer than Durkheim, and, as Mucchielli and Renneville show, a more precise statistician; he also lacked Durkheim's bias against subjectivity. Halbwachs's monograph *The Causes of Suicide* (1930) identified an existential loneliness that, if not entirely new, flourished in the growing towns and cities of nineteenth-century Europe and the countryside they engulfed.

Cities create opportunities for social and economic advancement, but they also create the conditions for exploitative relationships, swindles, romantic betrayals, fragile friendships, broken families, unstable jobs, and many other sources of despair. As European cities grew, so did a new class of people who were particularly prone to suicide, including abandoned lovers, lonely widowers, workers who'd lost their jobs, nobles shamed by some dishonorable act, gamblers who couldn't pay their debts, merchants who'd ruined themselves, heirs who'd squandered their fortunes, and others who'd suffered a common bitter fate: sudden exclusion from a cherished social community.

> They all see their social level lowered. They are to a certain extent declassed. But what does it mean to be declassed? It is to pass from a group that one knows, that esteems you, to

another that ignores you and whose appreciation one has no reason to hold. One then feels a void opening around oneself. Those who once surrounded you, with whom you had so many ideas in common, so many prejudices in common, with whom so many affinities brought you together because you found yourself in them as they found yourself in you, suddenly move away. You disappear from their concerns and their memory. Those among whom you find yourself understand neither your disorientation, nor your nostalgia and your regrets. Detached from the group by a sudden shock, you are incapable, or at least you believe yourself incapable of ever finding in another any support, nor anything to replace what you have lost.

Halbwachs quotes a passage from Johann Wolfgang von Goethe's 1774 novel, *The Sorrows of Young Werther*, which captures it better than just about anything I've ever read on the subject. Describing a girl who's been abandoned by a lover, Goethe writes:

Stunned, and almost out of her mind, she finds herself above an abyss; all around her is darkness; no way out, no consolation, no hope! The one person in whom she had found the center of her existence has left her. She does not see the wide world spread out before her or the many others who might replace her loss. She feels herself alone, abandoned by all—and blindly hunted into a corner by the terrible agony of her heart, she throws herself into the depths to drown all her anguish in the embrace of death.

20   In the midst of the nineteenth-century suicide crisis, the very meaning of the word "lonely" changed, from an adjective typically used to describe empty places and people who stood alone before God to one with the emotional and psychological connotations it has for us today. Suicidal despair, Halbwachs wrote, had been rarer in the past because traditional rural life was simpler and more predictable:

> We lived on the spot . . . adapted to each other, knowing each other too well to be frequently exposed to the clashes that occur when we move from one place, one situation, one profession, to another. Business carried less risk. Ambitions were less aroused, humiliations rarer. We thought and felt in common. Sorrows and troubles, instead of concentrating within the consciousness of this or that individual, dispersed and died out within the group.

What Halbwachs was describing was the transition from what German sociologist Ferdinand Tönnies called Gemeinschaft, or communities based on trust, mutual respect, and sharing of whatever material goods one had, to Gesellschaft, societies based largely on market transactions and political calculation in which ties of friendship and loyalty are relegated to private family life, and may not even reliably be found there. As far as I've been able to determine, and as the case studies in this book will show, wherever this transition has occurred, a suicide epidemic has followed swiftly behind.

But there is another ingredient too. As villagers shifted away from subsistence and small-scale farming to wage labor and trade, their intimate relationships became both more fragile and more precious. The extended family, which once formed a social mesh that supported everyone, waned in significance, and walls rose up around increasingly private and nuclearized families, usually dominated by a single, generally male breadwinner, upon whom everyone else in the family depended. If you felt your family didn't respect and care about you, you were in a new sort of trouble, not just because the community no longer offered you a livelihood, but because your whole identity was at stake. Modern capitalist society creates, in all of us, something of the double consciousness described by the great African American sociologist W. E. B. DuBois. When a modern person looks at a stranger, he wonders not only, as his villager ancestors did, "What can I do to help this person? And is he the kind of person who will help me?" but "What does that stranger see when he looks at me? What essence does he detect? A beauty or a beast? A success or a failure? A respectable person or a fool?"

The answer sometimes comes as a disappointment. In traditionally cohesive societies, this mattered less, because a person's worth was measured by what he did for others, and everyone was capable of contributing something. You might not be the best hunter, fisherman, storyteller, or drummer; you might not be the best grower of breadfruit or builder of igloos, but you still mattered. Only the greedy and selfish were looked down upon and excluded.

In modern societies, generosity still counts, but for far less than it used to. If others find us wanting—because of our looks, talents, graces, bank accounts, intelligence, or for whatever reason—we are alone with it, and must make sense of it, somehow.

22   For most of us, what makes modern life, with all its loneliness and insecurity, bearable are close relationships with people we count on to see and accept us for who we really are—whatever our flaws. Romantic rejection is exquisitely painful because we feel that that special quality within us, the thing that makes us lovable—and everyone has something—has either been unrecognized or, worse, seen and rejected. The pain of rejection by a parent or other close relative is even worse because it can make us feel as though no one could ever understand and sympathize with us. After all, they know us best of all. In the absence of an abstract sense of group belonging, interpersonal love, especially between parents and children and romantic partners, has become the main source of our psychological resilience, our ability to withstand the disappointments encountered in the outside world, just as the mutually reinforcing group gave strength to our ancestors fighting for survival on the plains, tundras, beaches, and forests of the past.

Love is not just a feeling; it's also a culture, which developed fairly recently, first in Western societies, and then around the world on the heels of capitalism, modernity, and individualism. It's no coincidence, the social philosopher Erich Fromm pointed out, that as modern ways of life displaced the traditional, cohesive village and clan, love poems, songs, and stories came to occupy the center of Western culture, displacing archaic tales of heroism and godliness. It's not that love was absent from the art of the ancient past, but as often as not, it was seen as a cause of calamity and human folly. Think of Helen of Troy, Dido and Aeneas, Adam and Eve. Then, more or less in lockstep with commercial culture and urbanization, love came to be seen as a force superior to the gods or God or honor or historic destiny.

The behavior of parents and spouses changed too. Until the 1800s, childrearing in England, for example, was seen as an exercise less in nurturing than in training for adulthood. Men who were fed up with their wives could sell them at markets or abandon them and marry someone else without divorcing. Infants who died weren't even listed in parish registers. Only in the nineteenth century did heartfelt observations of sons and daughters begin appearing regularly in the diaries of American and English mothers.

With the growth of markets and formal state institutions, people came to rely less on kinship networks for social welfare and trade and the family gradually shifted from an economic enterprise to a child-centered haven in a heartless world. The 1700s saw the first toy shops, women's magazines, popular childcare manuals, and family portraits. Christian churches, which had previously stressed family discipline and sometimes even the virtues of wife-beating, now promoted ideals of conjugal and parental love. Today, birthday parties, children's allowances, and Valentine's Day cards are symbols we use to assure each other that our most important relationships are real. Meanwhile, parenting manuals, happily-ever-after fairy tales, Hollywood movies, and the novels of Jane Austen, George Eliot, Charles Dickens, Barbara Cartland, Colleen Hoover, and countess others illustrate the enactment of love according to Western norms.

Premodern Europeans, as well as indigenous groups the world over, didn't need this culture because in the mutual aid communities of bygone days, you knew who you were and what you needed to do to gain the esteem of others: You had to pitch in for the group. You helped others and they helped you. That

24 was love, and according to accounts of anthropologists, it was everywhere, as ubiquitous as air. But when these groups modernized, in some cases very rapidly under the forces of capitalism and colonialism, the rules changed. Now it was unclear what the common goals were and what others were looking for in us. If they didn't like us, there wasn't a lot we could do about it. If the people we loved—our romantic partners, parents, and children—felt that way, it was intolerably painful because our hearts had nowhere to turn. Every rejection could now elicit devastating feelings of aloneness. "Who am I?" we are left to wonder. "Am I worth anything at all to anyone?"

Signifiers of love—birthday cards and so on—aren't enough. We need the confidence that our own feelings are understood. Some people, either because of the distortions of mental illness or because they really are lost and alone, simply don't have it.

Shortly before Jean died, she published a haunting oral history of five mid-twentieth-century Hollywood families, including her own. Her father, born in 1898 to poor Lithuanian immigrants, helped create the Jazz Age, and later, Hollywood itself out of the hardscrabble farmland of Southern California. When he was growing up, his family could barely feed itself; by age twenty-one, he owned a Stutz Bearcat car and a raccoon coat; at thirty-six, he was managing more than 90 percent of America's dance bands. Gangsters tried to kidnap him. Ronald Reagan was an honorary pallbearer.

Jean's people were the writers, directors, producers, and stars of films like *Gone with the Wind* and *Love Is a Many-Splendored Thing* that have touched the hearts of countless people the world over; movie stars came to dinner at the family's vast hilltop mansion, and for the children, there were ponies, swimming pools, and lavish birthday parties. But there was also coldness, cruelty, and parental abandonment. Virtually every family profiled in Jean's book is affected by suicide. One neglected child "falls" from the roof of a building; another shoots himself; others succumb to the slow suicide of alcoholism; an abandoned wife drinks battery fluid; another tries to drown herself.

The data isn't available to prove it, but early Hollywood families may also have experienced a suicide epidemic, and Jean's book, I now see, was a kind of suicide note. Less a cautionary tale of the corrupting effects of wealth on the human personality, it reads like an account of ordinary people marooned in a surreal new world devoid of moral order. These were the people whose films offered us profound depictions of the culture of love, and yet so many of them couldn't seem to figure out what it is or how it's done in real life.

In her book, Jean writes little about her own upbringing. In retrospect, the omission makes me wonder: Perceived parental rejection in childhood may be the strongest suicide predictor of all. After a lifetime of reading suicide notes and speaking with suicidal people, Edwin Shneidman found that in nearly every case, they'd been haunted by "the loss of childhood's special joys," because their inborn need for love, respect, dignity, and attention had been "trampled on and frustrated by malicious, preoccupied or obtuse adults"—many of whom had probably been trampled on themselves when they were children. These early miseries echo through the years, Shneidman laments, deepening the wounds of every subsequent rejection and disappointment.

26   In the book, Jean's mother is sketched only briefly. Jean's childhood friend, the writer Gore Vidal, remarks, "The early dawn" would see their two mothers pouring the first martinis. Once, Jean didn't show up for a party where her mother had planned to show her off. Another young woman was there, also from a prominent Los Angeles family. Jean's mother introduced the young guest to the others as Jean. This was Hollywood, where someone could always be found to play the part you thought was yours.

Jean smiled painfully when I told her how much I liked her book, but refused to say anything more about it. Since she died, I've been trying to understand what makes some groups of people vulnerable to epidemics of suicide, and also what has helped them endure.

The Inuit:
The Highest Suicide
Rate in the World

Sam was making toast at around 6:00 a.m. when he noticed the slit of light beneath the bathroom door. Minutes passed, but no one seemed to be moving inside and no one came out. In a dream that night, his wife, Maureen, had heard someone calling their daughter Sarah's name. She knew what had happened as soon as Sam shook her awake.

Clinging to the wall, Maureen approached the bathroom. And then she saw Sarah hanging in the shower stall, dead at age seventeen. The girl, Maureen told me, had just come back from visiting relatives in another village and had spent the previous afternoon sorting through clothes she wanted to give away. Then the family settled down to butcher and eat a seal—raw, in the traditional Inuit way—on a piece of cardboard on the sitting room floor. Afterward, Sarah put on some makeup and went out. She'd just broken up with an older boyfriend who her parents did not approve of, but they'd had so many fights about it that Maureen didn't dare ask where she was going.

28   If Nunavut, the semi-autonomous Canadian territory that is home to roughly 28,000 indigenous Inuit people, were an independent country, it would have the highest suicide rate in the world. The suicide rate in Greenland, whose population is mostly Inuit, is 85 per 100,000; next highest is Lithuania, at 32 per 100,000. Nunavut's rate is 100 per 100,000, ten times higher than the rest of Canada and seven times higher than the US. When I visited Nunavut's capital, Iqaluit, in July, virtually every Inuit I met had lost at least one relative to suicide, and some recounted as many as five or six family suicides, plus those of friends, coworkers, and other acquaintances. Three people in my small circle of contacts lost someone close to them to suicide during my nine-day visit. Acquaintances would direct my attention to passersby on the street: "his older brother too," "his son." Almost one-third of Nunavut Inuit have attempted suicide, and most Inuit I met confided, without my asking, that they had done so at least once.

The origins of the suicide crisis in Nunavut can be traced to the mid-twentieth century, when these traditionally nomadic people moved off the land into towns. Until then, suicide was rare, and among young people, almost unknown. Town life was safer and more comfortable than life on the land, but the transition nearly shattered the culture of these tough, inventive people, along with their sense of who they were.

The Inuit migrated across the Bering Land Bridge from what is now Siberia around 16,000 years ago and in 1000 CE settled in what is now northeastern Canada. There, in the long winter darkness, the wind is so strong that blowing snow can draw blood from exposed skin, and the windchill temperature

sometimes plunges to −60° Fahrenheit. In summer, swarms of
mosquitoes can exsanguinate a caribou. Nothing grows except
berries, moss, and wildflowers, so the Inuit hunted seals, fish,
birds, polar bears, caribou, walruses, and whales. The Inuit
made houses from snow, skins, and moss, and wore fur clothes
sewn with sinew threads and needles carved from slivers of wal-
rus bone. They constructed dogsleds from antlers, with frozen fish wrapped in sealskin for runners, and ingenious eye-slit
goggles carved from caribou bones that protected them from the
blinding light reflected off the snow.

But the Inuits' most remarkable innovation may have been
in the realm of interpersonal relations. Until the arrival of missionaries in the late nineteenth century, they had no written
language, so all that is known of their culture before that time
comes from the observations of explorers and ethnographers
and the memories of older Inuit passed down through generations. These sources all agree that traditional Inuit society was
remarkably peaceful and largely free of discord.

"The different families appear always to live on good terms
with each other," wrote British explorer Sir William Edward
Parry, who spent eight months among the Inuit of Baffin Island
beginning in 1821. "The more turbulent passions which . . .
usually create so much havoc in the world, seem to be very seldom excited in the breasts of these people." Inuit children were
"affectionate, attached, and obedient," concurred Sir John Ross,
who arrived a few years later. "These people had attained that
perfection of domestic happiness which is so rarely found
anywhere."

If conflicts did arise, wrongdoers were sometimes killed to
protect the rest of the group. But elders made sincere efforts at

30   reconciliation first; if that didn't work, singing duels might be organized in which the disaffected parties defused tension by making fun of each other. Violence tended to be carefully considered in advance as a group decision, and used only as a last resort against those whose behavior endangered others.

Today, homicide, domestic violence, child abuse, vandalism, and alcoholism—as well as suicide—are tragically common among the Inuit. The weekend I arrived in Iqaluit, population 7,740, there was one murder and four fires, three of which had been set deliberately. A brawling couple, the man bleeding from his head, the woman hurling abuse at him, nearly reeled into me in a shop one afternoon. A teacher told me that angry children have been known to throw furniture around the classroom. According to anthropologist Willem Rasing, over half the population uses drugs, mostly marijuana, but also stronger substances, including anything sniffable: starter fluid, spray paint, nail polish, and gasoline.

Most Inuit are law-abiding shop assistants, artists, government officials, and so on, but the relatively high rates of violence against property, the self, and others perpetrated by a minority of them raise urgent questions about what befell this once strong and stable culture. Everyone agrees the trouble started in the 1950s, but there is considerable disagreement between the Canadian government and most Inuit as to exactly what happened and why. The Canadian government maintains that during the late nineteenth century, many Inuit came to depend in part on money from the fur trade, which enabled them to purchase commodities like flour, sugar, guns, and knives, even as they maintained their traditional nomadic lifestyle. The collapse of the fur trade during the Great Depression, along with a cyclical decline in game populations, led to hardship, including cases of hunger and starvation. Many Inuit also succumbed to tuberculosis, measles, and other infectious diseases introduced by contact with whites. Patients were airlifted to hospitals in southern Canada, where they were sometimes confined for months or years and had no contact with their families. Some never returned.

The Canadian public demanded humanitarian intervention, so in the 1950s and 1960s, the government constructed houses for the Inuit around the old trading posts. Clinics, schools, government offices, and shops were built, and some Inuit were employed as fishermen, clerks, cleaners, garbage collectors, and cooks; others received state welfare. By the late 1960s, virtually all Inuit had moved into towns.

Most Inuit look back very differently on this period. Their version begins shortly after World War II, when the US and Canada jointly established a line of radar stations across the Arctic in order to spy on the Soviets and monitor the skies for potential attacks via the North Pole. The Canadian government, keen to prevent the US from claiming sovereignty over this mineral- and natural gas—rich area, hastily established towns and forced the Inuit to settle in them. Older Inuit told me they remember armed police officers arriving at their camps unannounced and ordering everyone to leave. Sled dogs—even healthy ones—were slaughtered before their owners' eyes. "One family I know was sitting in their house in town when the RCMP [Royal Canadian Mounted Police] showed up and shot all their dogs," said Alice, who collected testimonies for an Inuit-initiated inquiry into the dog killings. "They even shot under the crawlspace, right below where the family was sitting."

32   The government concedes that thousands of Inuit children, some as young as five, were sent to boarding, or "residential," schools, where they were cut off from their families, given Christian names and ID numbers, punished for speaking their native Inuktitut language, required to wear Western clothes, and taught a Canadian curriculum that had no relevance to the world they'd been born into. Many were also beaten and raped by their teachers. Some went to the schools willingly, but many reluctant parents, informed that if they didn't send their children off they'd be denied government welfare benefits or credit from fur traders, surrendered them in tears.

Memories of these horrors haunt the lives of older Inuit today. One elder told me she was terrified of the teachers at her residential school. When she was in third grade, she was asked to write the answer to the problem 5 x 3 on the blackboard. "I hadn't even finished writing the number 12 when the teacher hit me so hard, I went flying across the room," she said. Then he hit her again. He only stopped when he saw her nose was bleeding.

Across Canada, some 150,000 First Nations, Inuit, and other aboriginal children attended residential schools. Some did well, but thousands died from disease and hunger, at a rate comparable to that of Canadian soldiers during World War II. The Canadian government has paid out over Can$3 billion in compensation to tens of thousands of former students who suffered sexual or serious physical abuse in the schools. In a 2015 report by a truth and reconciliation commission that examined abuses in the residential schools, Canadian officials admitted that the schools' effect on aboriginal cultures amounted to a form of genocide.

Inuit suicides remained rare while the worst of these abuses were taking place. According to the University of Saskatchewan researcher Jack Hicks, who prepared a report on the subject, during the 1960s the number of deaths by suicide was low in what is now Nunavut (once part of Canada's Northwest Territories, it officially became a separate territory in 1999), and was almost unknown among young people. But as the children of the people who lived through the move to the towns became teenagers in the 1980s, they began taking their own lives in huge numbers. In 1973, the suicide rate in Nunavut was 11 per 100,000 people, about the same as in the rest of Canada. By 1986, it had quadrupled, and by 1997 it had increased tenfold, to 100 per 100,000. Most of the increase was due to a rise in suicide among young people aged fifteen to twenty-four. In the early 2000s, the suicide rate in this group peaked at 458 per 100,000; since then it has fallen to around 270 per 100,000. During this period, the suicide rate among young Canadians in general remained below 20 per 100,000.

How is trauma transmitted from one generation to the next? How do our experiences affect the emotional lives of our children and grandchildren? The answer isn't obvious. As discussed in the introduction, during the past century, American descendants of enslaved Africans have taken their own lives at lower rates than US whites, and the children of Jews in Nazi-occupied Europe were no more likely to die by suicide than the children of Jews who lived outside Nazi-occupied lands at the time.

Certain groups, however, including Australian aborigines, New Zealand Maoris, and the Inuit of Alaska, Greenland, and Canada, along with some other Native American groups, are particularly prone to youth suicide, generation after generation.

34   People in every society take their own lives for myriad reasons,
and it's obviously risky to generalize. Certainly, mental health
issues such as depression, anxiety, substance abuse, and schizophrenia are important risk factors for suicide everywhere. But
such disorders often have social causes, and it's worth asking if
there are any that might be responsible for the high suicide rates
among these peoples.

One clue is that virtually all these groups lived until recently
in small communities of one or a few extended families and then
underwent a forced, rapid, and harrowing transition to modern
life. Mastering technology—telephones, cars, computers, etc.—
was easy, but psychological and emotional adaptation has been
far more difficult. There have been several scholarly accounts of
this transition, but few offer the kind of detailed personal stories that might shed light on how the upheavals experienced by
one generation of Inuit might have led to mental turmoil in their
children and grandchildren.

For a deeper perspective on what might have happened, it's
helpful to turn to the anthropologist Jean Briggs's remarkable
1970 monograph, *Never in Anger: Portrait of an Eskimo Family*,
one of the last firsthand accounts of presettlement Inuit life.
Briggs suggests that the equanimity that so struck Parry and
the other explorers was produced by patterns of thought and
behavior, in particular consideration for others and a tendency
to privilege the welfare of the group over the self, that may have
been essential to Inuit survival on the land but could have made
them especially vulnerable to emotional difficulties once they
settled in towns.

In 1963, Briggs, then thirty-four, set out for Gjoa Haven, a
trading post in what is now Nunavut. Previous anthropologists

had documented Inuit material culture—how they hunted, built igloos, and made clothing—as well as their religious and cosmological beliefs. But Briggs was part of a school of anthropologists who maintained that, just as different cultures had different music, foods, and rituals, they also expressed different repertoires of emotion. For seventeen months, Briggs lived with a man named Inuttiaq and his wife and children, pitching a tent beside theirs in the summer and sharing their igloos in the winter. At first, she worried about living in such close quarters with people whose culture was so different from hers, but like other observers, she was quickly beguiled and moved by the tranquility of Inuit domestic life: "The human warmth and peacefulness of the household, and the uncanny sensitivity of its members to unspoken wishes, created an atmosphere in which the privacy of my tent came to seem in memory a barren thing."

This peaceful surface, Briggs would discover, was undergirded by a powerful system of emotional control and social regulation. Expressions of anger, shock, romantic ardor, and other strong feelings were all but absent from everyday life, except among very small children. One informant even denied that the Inuit language had a word for "hate"—although of course it does. Briggs's host family's oldest daughter was among the first children to attend a residential school. When she returned for the summer, she brought back horror stories of a "strange [white] world where people are always loud and angry . . . where they hit their children, let babies cry, kiss grown-ups, and make pets of dogs and cats."

Children learned early how to manage their feelings, through what Briggs describes as a process of emotional weight training.

36 Toddlers were indulged, doted on, and seldom disciplined, but they were also subject to joking questions from parents and other adults that must have been confusing and scary to them:

> Why don't you kill your baby brother?
> Why don't you die so I can have your nice new shirt?
> Where's your father? [to an adopted child]
> Your mother's going to die—look, she's cut her finger—do you want to come live with me?

An adult would never ask such questions when a child was upset, and would stop and offer a hug at the first signs of distress. Briggs interpreted these exchanges as immunization against the offhand insensitivity of others and life's ordinary misfortunes and disappointments. "Adults stimulate children to think by presenting them with emotionally powerful problems," she wrote. The goal was emotional strength and rationality. In a harsh environment, mutual understanding and trust are essential to survival. An unhappy person is a dangerous one.

As Briggs would soon learn the hard way, everyone was on guard against the slightest increase in the emotional temperature. Her hosts were fox hunters who traded with whites in a town several days away by dogsled from their winter camp. Fried bread made from store-bought flour was a great delicacy, and one day, as Briggs was preparing some with the others, a piece of dough slipped off her knife and fell into the fire.

"Damn!" she said under her breath.

Over the following days, weeks, and months, Briggs noticed a change in the family's behavior. They came to visit her tent less often and left quickly when they did. They seemed even

more solicitous than usual, as if she were afflicted with some 37
sort of disease. They made sure she was warm and had enough
to eat but didn't invite her on fishing trips.

Gradually, she realized that she was being ostracized, not
just for the fried bread incident, but for other flashes of irrita-
tion, such as when Inuttiaq insisted on leaving the igloo door-
way open, making it too cold for Briggs to type her field notes.
Imagine the shock of these polite, dignified people when some
RCMP officers killed their dogs and ordered them into the
settlements, when some residential schoolteachers abused
them, and other powerful *qallunaats*—as whites are known in
the Inuktitut language—insulted and patronized them. Many of
the residential school children, in particular, came back angry
and alienated. The emotional training they'd received as toddlers was no match for the arrogance, insensitivity, and stupid-
ity, let alone brutality, that they encountered in the *qallunaat*
world. With no language to describe their hurt and loneliness,
they turned away from their families.

The residential school student in the family Briggs lived
with avoided her parents and tormented her little sister, deliberately stepping on her toes, snatching her toys, and making her
cry. When asked to do something, she pretended to be deaf. As
adults, a great many of the former residential school children
resorted to alcohol to tame their emotional turmoil. Their children, raised in the 1970s and 1980s, largely escaped the residential schools, which were already being replaced with community
schools. But their parents had never managed to come to terms
with their own anger and grief, and were often drunk and violent. In this way, the first suicide generation was born, and their
children continue the trend.

38   Anthropologist Michael Kral interviewed dozens of young Inuit men who had attempted suicide. Most told him that they tried to take their own lives after a fight with a romantic partner. Coroner reports from the 1990s also found that some 70 percent of suicides occurred after a romantic breakup and another 20 percent occurred while awaiting trial for an alleged crime—mostly break-ins and marijuana use. These ordinary predicaments occur everywhere. Why are Inuit youth who experience them so much more likely to resort to suicide?

"The theory I have is that [Inuit] who commit suicide are doing it to protect the community," Bonnie, an Inuit government official, told me when I visited Iqaluit.

> When we lived in small groups, we had a contract for survival. You lived for the collective, not for yourself. We're in this together. Children are conditioned to be calm. If someone explodes, that person is a threat to everyone. Then [the one who exploded] thinks, "Everyone will be better off without me. I'm a problem because I can't handle my emotions." It's hard to get that out of your head, because we're conditioned not to be a burden to others.

A friend of Bonnie's had recently come to her in tears, saying he feared he might take his own life. He was one of the best young hunters in the community. He'd just caught a seal and left it in a small square in town, where others knew they could take some of the meat for free. In the old days, he'd have been seen as a hero, but in the dull, materialistic world of supermarkets and welfare checks, he realized with terrible loneliness that hunting was now just a hobby, with meaning only to himself.

There are no simple answers to the Nunavut suicide crisis. Some experts maintain that community activities such as
sports can help by increasing social cohesion. The penultimate
chapter of Michael Kral's *The Return of the Sun* describes a recreation center Kral helped establish with a group of young
Inuit in the town where he did his research. He claims that,
while it operated, the number of suicides there fell to zero. Data
from the coroner's office cited by Jack Hicks indicates that this
is not the case. Similarly, a 2005 ESPN feature claimed that
the number of teen suicides in the Nunavut town of Kugluktuk
fell to zero after a visiting teacher started a lacrosse team, but
there were twenty-one suicides among people aged thirteen
to fifty-six in Kugluktuk in the following decade. These communities are so small—average populations are around fifteen hundred each—that suicide rates may vary from year to
year just because of chance. A high-suicide community may
have no suicides at all for several years, creating a temporary
illusion of success, even when the long-term trend is stable or
increasing.

In 2017, the government of Nunavut launched a comprehensive suicide prevention strategy that includes mental health
services, early childhood programs, community awareness programs, anti-bullying programs, youth centers, housing assis-
tance, poverty reduction, crime and substance abuse prevention,
and many other initiatives. Such multifaceted approaches have
been shown to reduce suicides in other communities, such as
the White Mountain Apaches in the US, and there's every reason
to believe that Nunavut's new strategy will help too.

In 2018, the local radio station in Iqaluit broadcast a call-in
program on suicide. Alice, whose son Martin took his own life

40 that year, called in to say that the community needed more counselors, and if there weren't enough, then the people should just form their own support groups. "Talking is part of healing," she told me. "People have been quiet for too long." Alice herself had been sexually assaulted when she was seven—she didn't discuss the circumstances—and believes she would have become a drunk on the street if not for the counseling she eventually received in her late twenties.

Other listeners phoned in to say they supported Alice's idea. Elisapee Johnston, who works for the Embrace Life Council, a local NGO funded under the new suicide prevention strategy, was listening. She tracked Alice down, and the two women agreed to work together. In the spring of 2019, they launched a bereavement group that meets weekly at the Embrace Life Council's office in downtown Iqaluit. Anyone who's lost someone to suicide, or who is simply worried about it, is welcome.

"Young people really need coping skills," Alice insists, but getting people to turn up at meetings has been a challenge. "People come up and hug me on the street and say, 'Thank you, thank you for all that you are doing,' but only when they're drunk."

It's just not the Inuit way to talk about yourself. Another Inuit elder told me that when her family's dogs were killed, no one discussed it: "They must have been angry, but they didn't show it." For years, she'd taught elementary school but objected to elements of the Canadian curriculum. "I had to teach a kindergarten unit called 'All About Me.' In our culture, that age group is supposed to think about others." An anthropologist I met told me she'd struggled to collect Inuit testimonies about trauma that filled more than half a page. Such modesty and discretion is refreshing in these self-oriented, tell-all times, but if people won't talk about themselves, it's hard to see how they'll manage to make sense of their feelings.

In 2021, nearly one hundred young Inuit marched through the streets of Iqaluit to demand better mental health services, and although the suicide rate remains high, new government plans and increased funding have been forthcoming. The young activists can take heart from the experience of other traumatized groups, including African Americans and the descendants of Holocaust survivors, who, though disproportionately subject to some mental health problems, have relatively low suicide rates. What enables them to endure? It's worth noting that mourning, sharing experiences of personal suffering, and the ongoing search for a promised land are integral to the religions and cultures of both groups. So is the belief that anger is sometimes justified, and that living, hard as it may be sometimes, is also a form of defiance.

Sturm und Drang in Micronesia

Some five thousand years ago, seafarers set out from what is now Taiwan in wooden double-hulled canoes with sails woven from tree fronds. No one knows why they left, but they plied nearly the entire Pacific Ocean, navigating via the stars from Madagascar to Easter Island, settling what is now Micronesia beginning around 1500 BCE. There, they found thousands of tiny tropical islands lush with coconut and breadfruit trees and reefs shimmering with fish.

They built a society based on sharing and cooperation. There were no banks or money, and since fish and coconuts rot, it was impossible to accumulate wealth. What mattered were relationships, people you could rely on when your own luck ran out. Your lineage—your family, including parents, grandparents, uncles, aunts, cousins, children, and so on—were what made you you.

They say "we" all the time, where Americans would say "I" or "you," observed anthropologist Catherine Lutz, who spent a year on Ifaluk, one of the remotest and most traditional

Micronesian islands, in the 1980s. As a person without family or taro gardens, Lutz was seen as having special needs; people were constantly offering her food, teaching her words, patting her arm. They sat with her when she was sick and constantly reminded her to keep in the shade. Common names for women translated as "Love and desire," "Love and generosity," and "Love binding." In the West, explains Lutz, it's normal to get angry at someone for smoking without asking permission because he's polluting your personal airspace. In Micronesia, anger was only justified if the smoker didn't offer to share his cigarette with you—or if he took the chief's turtle without permission, walked by a group of elders without bending over in a traditional gesture of respect, or otherwise behaved selfishly. When Lutz once asked a group of Micronesian friends, "Do you want to go to the river to fetch water?" they lowered their heads in embarrassment. Only later did Lutz realize what she should have asked: "Do *we* want to go to the river?" In traditional Micronesian culture, decisions aren't made by individuals.

It was as if, she theorized, they had no sense of self inside, distinct from the public one. "Absent is the notion that . . . one should 'know oneself'" or even could do so "outside of the moral or social constraints that sometimes make introspection necessary."

"Humanity [in Micronesia] is one viscous mass," wrote another American observer. "Each individual, no matter who she is, or what she can do, blends in with the group so effortlessly that sometimes she seems to have no soul of her own," said another.

The idea that anyone would want to be alone, even for a short while, was inconceivable. In the old days, twenty people

44 might occupy a single one-room grass-thatched dwelling, but even after houses with multiple rooms were built in the 1960s, five or six people would pile in to sleep in each one. In *Making Sense of Micronesia*, his insightful portrait of life on the islands, American-born Jesuit priest Francis Hezel recounts the story of a Peace Corps volunteer who went to the beach one day to write in his journal. By and by, he looked up and saw two children from his host family staring at him. They'd been sent by their mother to check on him because, in her mind, only a suicidal person would wander off like that.

Fr. Hezel grew accustomed to the eyes of little children peering through the windows of his house every morning, and to students who, sensitive to the feelings of less able classmates, were reluctant to answer questions even when they could. What Hezel didn't know was that he'd arrived just in time to witness a massive experiment in international development that would have grave psychological consequences for these gentle people.

The Japanese launched the attack on Pearl Harbor from Micronesia, but since 1947, it had been a United Nations Trust Territory under US administration. During the 1950s, the Pentagon used some of the islands to test hydrogen bombs—the waste is still stored on one of them—and to house a CIA training school for anti-communist spies. But with the Vietnam War looming, the islands' people were now on Washington's radar. Guam, the largest island in the region, would serve as a hub for B-52s, making the winning of Micronesian hearts and minds a matter of national security. So, the Kennedy administration launched what may be the most ambitious economic and social development program ever attempted. It's aim was to bring the territory's roughly one hundred thousand people into the twentieth century.

Almost overnight, the economy changed from one based on fishing, subsistence agriculture, and dried coconut exports to one based on jobs and cash. By the 1980s, 90 percent of all food consumed on the islands was imported, concrete houses and tin roofs had replaced the grass huts of bygone days, and the sons and daughters of fishermen had become office and construction workers. Old missionary schools and hospitals were upgraded and new ones built. Per capita income quadrupled in just thirty years as the civil service expanded and construction and trade increased. It was, anthropologist Glen Petersen explained to me, a kind of welfare state utopia, or upside-down colonialism, where no one paid taxes and hundreds of millions of dollars—billions in today's money—poured into Micronesia's treasury as if from the gods.

Fr. Hezel had been living in Micronesia on and off for about a decade when he realized the modernization program was having disastrous effects on community life. Theft, assault, and homicide, all but unknown in the past, soared, as did alcohol consumption. Once-pristine beaches were now carpeted with beer cans, and boys as young as eight played at being drunks—reeling through the streets shouting and pretending to guzzle from empty bottles. Some Micronesians wondered whether accepting American foreign aid had meant selling their souls to the devil.

The most heartbreaking aspect of this social catastrophe was the suicide rate, which rose sixfold between 1960 and 1983. On one survey, half the population said they'd attempted suicide at one time or another. Fr. Hezel could see it in his students' eyes. "They're such beautiful people," he told journalist David Nevin, "the kids, you know, they smile and they're so open and warm and joyous, until they're about fifteen, and then something seems to close down on them. Some light goes out."

Over the next fifty years, Hezel, along with anthropologist Donald Rubinstein, documented virtually every suicide on the islands—more than fifteen hundred in all—to see if they could identify any patterns.

The vast majority of suicides were young men, between the ages of fifteen and twenty-five. Very few suffered from mental illnesses of any kind; nor had they been physically ill. Unlike Japanese youths, young Micronesians didn't take their own lives when they flunked out of school or lost a job. In fact, suicides were slightly more common among those who were in school or working, compared to unemployed dropouts. Nor was this a case of simple Durkheimian urban dislocation. Although almost no suicides occurred on the outer islands where people still lived more or less according to the old ways, suicide rates in the larger town centers were also relatively low. The hot spots were in the periphery, Micronesia's new suburbia, where men commuted to the towns and larger islands for construction or civil service jobs.

The trigger was almost always some domestic dispute that seems trivial on the face of it—most often with the victim's father or older brother, but sometimes his wife or girlfriend. A great many suicides followed a father's refusal of a request for a small amount of money, a new shirt, or permission to borrow the family car. One boy who stayed out too late so feared his father's reaction that he hanged himself on the way home. Another killed himself after a fight over

a flashlight. Another took his own life after learning that his
father, who had just refused him five dollars, had given his
older brother ten.

Sima's case was typical. One morning, his father told Sima
to meet him at a certain breadfruit tree, and to bring a knife to
cut down the fruit. Sima searched the neighborhood for a knife,
but couldn't find one and, on top of that, was late. "Get out of
here, and go find somewhere else to live!" his father shouted at
him when he finally turned up.

Sima went home and hanged himself, leaving behind the
following note:

> My life is coming to an end at this time. Now today is a day
> of sorrow for myself, also a day of suffering for me. But it
> is a day of celebration for Papa. Today Papa sent me away.
> Thank you for loving me so little. [signed] Sima
> Give my farewell to Mama. Mama, you won't have any
> more frustration or trouble from your boy. Much love from
> Sima.

According to Hezel, severe child abuse and neglect, though
not uncommon in Micronesia, were not usually present in the
families of the young people who took their own lives. But ordinary family quarrels were absolutely devastating, especially for
young men. People laughed, he writes, when talking about getting robbed, having their houses blown down by a typhoon, and
even when recalling being bombed and tortured by Japanese
occupiers during World War II. But when someone close to
them died, or when they fought with a relative, nothing could be
more serious.

He may fail out of school, his business may go under, his boat may sink and his house be destroyed by a typhoon, and he may lose his government job; but he will not be driven to despair provided that he is assured of the love and respect of those closest to him. When this is withdrawn, he senses that he is a failure: it no longer matters to anyone whether he lives or dies. At this point almost any incident, however insignificant, may serve to confirm this dreadful latent feeling and provide the necessary impetus to commit the final deed.

Hezel appears to have been witnessing the birth pangs of individualism, the terrifying realization that, in modern societies, we are really, truly, alone, and even our parents may not care about our feelings. The young were most affected because this is when the search for self is most urgent.

Early-twentieth-century psychologists called it *Sturm und Drang*—or Storm and Stress—a reference to the late-eighteenth-century artistic period, with its paintings of rain clouds and shipwrecks, and novels in which young characters are so overwhelmed by their emotions they can't bear to be alive. American psychologist Stanley Hall produced the first comprehensive account of it in his 1904 volume *The Psychology of Adolescence*, in which he likens this period of life to a second birth, this time for the emotions, rather than the body.

At about age thirteen, Hall wrote, young people began to exhibit what George Eliot referred to as "volcanic upheavings of imprisoned passions." They rebel, take risks, and experience wild swings of ecstasy, sorrow, fear, and rage. Culling from the biographies of writers and diarists, Hall recounts how, as adolescents, they told fantastic lies (Leo Tolstoy), wept for no reason (Jean Jacques Rousseau), climbed trees at midnight (Louisa May Alcott), conversed with flowers (Frances Hodgson Burnett), accidentally, while chopping wood, cut off a finger when a girl walked by (Jacob Riis), obsessed over their souls and their loves (everybody), had revelations, fell into inexplicable despair, joined revolutions, alternated between worshipping their teachers and believing them to be hypocrites, fantasized about marrying Satan, declaimed poetry on lonely hills at sunset, built altars to imaginary gods, saw ghosts, bore witness to the celestial correspondence of the universe, and lay in the grass wishing they were dead.

Hall's book set off a fierce debate. Was adolescent *Sturm und Drang* universal, as psychoanalysts like Anna Freud—Sigmund's daughter—maintained? Or was it a product of modernity? The following decades were the heyday of cultural anthropology. Researchers fanned out across the globe to study the customs of so-called primitive peoples in order to discern whether there were larger patterns common to all humanity. It soon became clear that youths in unmodernized societies largely escaped the angst, confusion, and misery of adolescence. Their bodies changed, they started experimenting with sex and took on new roles in the family and community, but most did so in trauma-free ways. This was true not only in Micronesia, but also in Samoa, famously portrayed by the great cultural anthropologist Margaret Mead, and in more than 180 other communities around the world, according to an exhaustive 1991 review carried out by Alice Schlegel and Herbert Barry III.

So, what was it about Micronesia's warp speed modernization program that sparked an epidemic of adolescent Storm and

50   Stress? American money, Hezel and others theorized, had radically altered the dynamics of family life.

      In the past, extended families comprising thirty or forty
people formed cooperative enterprises, in which everyone,
even children as young as three or four, played a constructive
role—gathering coconuts, helping to build canoes, fishing in
the lagoon, caring for younger kids, and so on. With this came a
sense of equality between parents and children. Fathers, in particular, had been more like friends or kindly teachers than the
owners of their children. In the mostly matrilineal societies of
Micronesia, your maternal uncle was the real head of the family,
and if a young person had a conflict with his father, he'd normally go off to his uncle's house, or to some other elder in the
lineage, until his parents coaxed him to come home, at which
point everything would return to normal. Micronesians have a
word for the emotions evoked in such cases: Amwunumwun—a
kind of hurt retreat. It's a form of anger, but its purpose isn't to
punish; it's to bring a relationship back into alignment by signaling that the offender has violated the moral code of together-
ness by ignoring the sufferer's feelings.

      The Americanization program made people richer in some
ways, but family life changed radically, and not for the better. As
families came to depend more on the earnings of male bread-
winners, they cooperated with each other less. In the past, when
one household borrowed from another, no one kept track of who
owed what to whom; now, exact repayment was expected. Canned
mackerel and imported rice became the new staple foods; women
stopped fishing and stayed home cooking and cleaning and looking after kids, relying, much as 1950s American housewives did,
almost exclusively on money from a husband's pocket. Men still

farmed, but now they put inordinate energy into prestige crops, especially yams, which in Micronesia can grow to over two hundred pounds. Giving a large yam to the chief came to be the ultimate masculine achievement. Meanwhile, growing numbers of children in this confused new patriarchy began to succumb to malnutrition, even though there were no food shortages.

Some fathers, annoyed by wives and children who now pestered them for money all the time, became impatient, and even tyrannical. While older girls could find a role for themselves helping their mothers, older boys and young men found themselves adrift and without purpose. When they quarreled with their fathers over money, they had nowhere to turn because the lineage system had broken down and their uncles had their own families to deal with.

It's not that fathers didn't love their troubled sons; many, or even most of them, probably did. But they didn't have a script to express it, or even know that one existed. Like that of the Inuit and other suicide-prone societies, traditional Micronesian culture is stoic; people seldom psychologize their personal problems or express emotions openly. Micronesian children learn from earliest childhood to suppress their feelings with resolute positivity, not all that different from the can-do, upbeat attitude of soldiers. Gatherings among friends may be rowdy, but family occasions are solemn and ritualized. When Fr. Hezel once asked a Micronesian Jesuit novice when he knew his father loved him, the young man recalled that they'd been out fishing when his father grunted at him. "Then I knew."

Love is part of our biology; just about every human, and perhaps every mammal and maybe even every bird, feels it at one time or another. But in traditionally cohesive human

52   societies like that of the Micronesians, it's rarely spoken of, so
young people in the throes of the Americanization program had
no idea if their parents loved them or not. Small gifts and allowances acquired inordinate significance because they provided
some glimpse of what was going on in their parents' hearts. For
those who received nothing, the darkness could be impossible
to bear. These young Micronesians might be seen as pioneers of
a sort, on a mission they had not chosen, into the world of the
modern self. Some wouldn't survive the journey.

In Western societies, love rituals help hold the modern
family together. Americans, for example, now fork over some
$85 billion annually on children's allowances. These payments
are not in exchange for labor—some kids do chores, but these
tend to be character building, not to support the household.
Micronesian parents didn't understand how the denial of such
gifts could convey a lack of love, and because contradicting or
interrupting a parent was unthinkable, there was no way for a
young Micronesian to explain this, except by running away—or,
if there was nowhere to run, taking his own life.

Or, in some cases, going on an emotional rampage. On typical warm weekend nights at the height of the youth suicide crisis in the 1980s, young men across Micronesia would gather in
bars or in the bush and drink until they were blitzed out of their
minds. Occasionally, one of them would fill the night air with
war cries as he and his comrades wove through the streets kick-
ing down doors kung-fu style, trashing houses, attacking police,
and even, occasionally, killing someone. Entire villages would
come out to witness the mayhem.

Anthropologist Mac Marshall came to see these rampages
as cultural rituals, enactments of feelings young Micronesians

were unable to express when sober, not unlike the trancelike ritual dances of Africa, with their angry masks and wild animal costumes. As with suicides, the rampages were virtually always triggered by some painful interpersonal conflict—rejection by a lover or, more often, a scolding by a close family member, usually a father or an older brother. The drunks and the suicidal kids seemed to be responding in different ways to the same thing: the feeling of living in an intensely threatening emotional landscape for which their culture left them unprepared.

Few, if any, of the young rampagers were alcoholics; they didn't drink all the time—just on rampage evenings, when unleashing feelings of hurt and anger was made socially permissible because they were assumed to be drunk and out of control. On at least two occasions, a young rampager, noticing Marshall in the crowd of onlookers, walked over to him like an actor breaking character, and attempted to explain, in English, what was going on. Sometimes a rampage would end in suicide, but most suicides weren't rampage-related. "It's the quiet ones we lose," says a social worker in a short film about suicide on the islands. "It's the dutiful ones, not the hell-raisers," Hezel confirmed to me.

During World War I, anthropologist Bronisław Malinowski found himself stranded on the Trobriand Islands, a tiny archipelago roughly a thousand miles northeast of Australia, whose people share many of the customs of the Micronesians. Unable to return to graduate school in Britain because it and his native Poland were at war, Malinowski immersed himself in the lives of the Trobriand islanders. He was miserable much of the time. He feared he had tuberculosis, felt constantly on the verge of

54   throwing up, and was so annoyed and frustrated with the natives that he even considered suicide. But he saw something. Until then, many anthropologists still viewed non-European peoples as evolutionary relics, savages trapped in some pre-civilized stage. Studying their rituals, customs, and sexuality was seen as a way of exploring the white European past before order, civilization, and reason supposedly prevailed.

But Malinowski found that the Trobrianders had a highly organized society, with rules and customs that differed in detail from those of Europeans, but had the same overall purpose. He likened societies to bodies and cultural practices to organs—livers, kidneys, and so on—that helped individuals manage their emotional reactions to the outside world. Funerals help us deal with grief; athletic contests help us understand joy and humiliation. "We develop the capacity to feel true awe in church," wrote anthropologist Clifford Geertz, who described culture in much the same way. "A child counts on his fingers before he counts 'in his head'; he feels love on his skin before he feels it 'in his heart.'"

In the fierce headwinds of the modern money-based economy, recent generations of Micronesians, like the Inuit and presumably other suicide-affected indigenous societies, are being forced to search for new cultural faculties to help maintain emotional equilibrium—something no society has yet perfectly achieved.

While researching the Micronesians, I read Goethe's late-eighteenth-century *Sturm und Drang* novel *The Sorrows of Young Werther*, in which the hero falls hopelessly in love with a young woman who's engaged to someone else. He manages to pull himself away and get a job, but then screws that up, returns to

the now married young woman, and throws himself at her feet,
whereupon she rejects him. Realizing the situation is hopeless,
he goes home and shoots himself.

In his forward to the 1971 edition of the book, the preeminent English love poet W. H. Auden dismisses young Werther as "a complete egoist, a spoiled brat, incapable of love because he cares for nobody and nothing but himself and having his way at whatever cost to others." What Auden fails to explain is why, despite Werther's evident flaws, the book remains in print 250 years after it was written. Werther is asking what we are all asking—most acutely when young, but really throughout life: Who will love me? Who will respect me? Who will understand me? These are the very questions young Micronesians would ask themselves two centuries later. The lineage system and the customs and rituals of survival and everyday life once offered young Micronesians an answer. Without this, their souls were like open wounds.

Russia's Traumatic Transition

Boris Yeltsin was so depressed he could barely follow a conversation. Upon taking over as Russia's first post-communist president in 1991, he'd launched a radical experiment: to transform, at breakneck speed, the Soviet planned economy into a capitalist, market-based one. Now, little more than a year later, he lay awake all night, wracked with headaches and insomnia, wondering whether he'd made a terrible mistake.

Change had been desperately needed. Under the Soviets, the government controlled prices and wages and state bureaucrats told factories what to produce based on estimates of how many Russians were expected to need cars, toothbrushes, platform shoes, or whatever. But nothing worked. There were hours-long supermarket lines, tons of fish rotted onshore while officials in Moscow tried to figure out what to do with them, and everything seemed to be exploding in a bonfire of quality control issues, from gas pipelines to the Chernobyl nuclear power plant to Russian TV sets—the leading cause of house fires in the country.

At a stroke, Yeltsin relaxed state control of the economy and
encouraged foreign trade—initiatives begun under his prede-
cessor, Mikhail Gorbachev. He then ordered the privatization
of over one hundred thousand state-owned factories, mines,
media houses, energy companies, and other firms.

He did this in the absence of a modern legal framework for
trade and finance, or an adequate state infrastructure to enforce
whatever laws did exist. The result, in the short term anyway, was chaos. The ruble collapsed and the economy shrank
at one point to the size of that of the United States in 1897. By
1996, a third of Russians would be living on less than $4 a day—
considered the level of subsistence. On city streets, desperate
people hawked family heirlooms, factory castoffs, and even their
shoes; poor people survived on potato peelings and chopped
down trees in city parks for firewood.

But some did well in the mayhem. Insiders snapped up
newly privatized companies at a tiny fraction of their true
value and then, rather than modernizing them, fired everyone and sold off the machinery for scrap. According to Stephen
Handelman, who chronicled Russian organized crime during
the early 1990s, half a million dollars' worth of metal from
decommissioned Russian factories, along with untold amounts
of weapons-grade uranium from Russian military installations,
was being smuggled out of the country every day. By 1994, some
four thousand criminal gangs controlled nearly half of all retail
trade in the country. Hit men murdered journalists, legislators,
and bankers and burned down rival businesses. Forty thousand
Russians were killed each year during the 1990s, and another
seventy thousand disappeared. The police, barely able to survive
on their rapidly diminishing salaries, sometimes had to pursue

58 criminals by bus. Even gangsters complained to Handelman about the lawlessness.

Before entering politics, Yeltsin had been a civil engineer, construction manager, and local government official. He knew how to tear things down and build something new. But as he drove to work in the morning, past kiosks burned out by gangland enforcers, drunks lying face down in the snow, old people rummaging through garbage cans, and long lines of people trying to get their money out of savings banks, he realized he'd never faced a problem like this.

Russia's politics were as chaotic as its economy. After a particularly grueling parliamentary session in December 1992, when legislators denounced him in speech after speech as a tyrannical buffoon, a drunk, and a puppet of American bankers, he came home, took one look at his wife and children, who'd also been complaining about the problems they saw all around them, and went straight to the *banya*—or household sauna. He locked the door, lay down on his back, and closed his eyes. Dark thoughts, he later wrote, swirled in his head. Eventually, a bodyguard managed to open the door and convince him to come out.

But his mental state did not improve. The parliamentary opposition, allied to a cadre of KGB spies and corrupt civil servants whom Yeltsin had fired, was preparing to impeach him. They organized gangs to wreak havoc around the city, and armies of babushkas to march on the main TV station waving photographs of Stalin. In March 1993, Yeltsin drew a pistol from a cabinet in his office and held it to his own head. Fortunately, the same bodyguard who'd rescued him from the *banya* had known about the gun, and arranged for the Kremlin chef to boil the cartridges. It would not have fired even if his aides had failed

to talk him back from the brink. But something was clearly very
wrong with Russia's head of state, and it was afflicting millions
of other Russians as well.

Around this time, I was studying public health at the London
School of Hygiene and Tropical Medicine. The school's 1920s
building, decorated with bronze tsetse flies, bedbugs, fleas,
ticks, and lice, was staffed mainly by experts in infectious diseases. But one day, about halfway through the fall semester, an
epidemiologist named David Leon gave a lecture about Russia,
where a different kind of plague was underway. Between 1989
and 1994, male life expectancy fell by six years—a mortality
effect similar, relatively speaking, to that of the US Civil War.
But in this case, nearly all the casualties were self-inflicted.
Suicides doubled among middle-aged men, who were now six
times as likely as middle-aged American men to take their own
lives. Alcohol-related deaths quintupled, not, for the most part,
due to chronic illnesses like liver cirrhosis that develop over
years, but from acute alcohol poisoning, which kills more or less
instantly. A little alcohol tickles the brain, but a lot—say two
or three bottles of vodka at a sitting—can shut it down completely. Heart-disease deaths also surged during this time, but
unlike Western cardiac patients, many Russian ones lacked
signs of blocked arteries or plaque upon autopsy. These deaths
were probably alcohol-related, too, since large amounts of alcohol can also shut down the heart.

Suicide and alcoholism are hard to disentangle. Even more
than other addictions, alcoholism is a huge risk factor for suicide, second only to depression. In the US, severe alcoholics are
roughly a hundred times more likely to take their own lives than

60   non-mentally ill controls. In 1990s Russia, nearly half of all working-age male suicides were heavy alcohol users.

In the years after Leon's findings were published, two schools of thought emerged about what was causing this plague of self-destructive behavior. One group, which I'll call the "overly-rapid-transition-to-capitalism-blamers," attributed it to the drastic nature of Russia's economic reforms. Mortality had actually fallen in other Eastern European post-communist states like Belarus and Poland, where the reforms had been more gradual, avoiding spikes in crime and unemployment. In their 2013 book, *The Body Economic*, public health experts David Stuckler and Sanjay Basu maintain that the Russian people were in the grip of an epidemic of despair brought about by factory closures, the removal of state subsidies and job guarantees, and the resulting poverty, loneliness, and boredom. "I can't explain it," an unemployed alcoholic named Vladimir told a journalist when asked why he was binge-drinking perfume—popular because it was cheaper than vodka. "I have a home. But I have nothing to do."

Other scholars, whom I'll call the "legacy-of-communism-blamers," maintained that what looked like a surge in mortality coincident with the transition was really the continuation of a centuries-long cultural trend. According to this hypothesis, Russian Slavs were originally a nomadic people who had been forcibly settled over centuries by an increasingly powerful feudal aristocratic state. The Russian lands are poorly suited to agriculture, and the growing season in much of the country is vanishingly short. The aristocracy nevertheless prospered on the labor of millions of oppressed serfs and peasants, who developed a culture of endurance, passivity, and resignation, along with a tendency to salve despair with alcohol, and in

extreme cases, suicide. This was adaptive under the Soviets—
who could be just as cruel and repressive as the czars. When
the boot was finally lifted during the late 1980s and '90s, what
looked like freedom to Western observers was experienced
by Russians as existential chaos, and they retreated from the
demands and responsibilities of capitalism into old patterns of
despair and alcohol-induced psychological stasis.

The legacy-of-communism-blamers did seem to have
history on their side. Russia's alcohol problem was not
new. Sixteenth- and seventeenth-century travelers' tales—
exaggerated, but no doubt containing a grain of truth—describe
the peasants, monks, and czars as more or less permanently
drunk. When Lenin attempted to limit alcohol production in the
1920s, a thousand-strong crowd outside one liquor store had
to be dispersed with machine guns. When Mikhail Gorbachev
tried again during the 1980s, illegal stills turned up in factories, Young Pioneers clubs, daycare centers, alcohol rehab centers, and in a third of private homes in some areas. When all else
failed, people drank not only perfume but also shoe polish and
printer's ink. Ground crews reportedly drank the de-icing fluid
in airplanes, and the MIG-25 fighter jet, whose braking system required half a ton of alcohol, became known as the "flying
restaurant."

The overly-rapid-transition-to-capitalism-blamers didn't
deny that Russians had always been drinkers; it's just that what
happened in the early 1990s was like nothing epidemiologists—
or anyone—had ever seen before. By 1993, Russian men were
consuming, on average, a bottle of vodka every two days.
Historian Stephen White writes that in some towns, half the
male population were alcoholics. Apartment building stairwells

62 and public toilets turned into drinking dens. "If you tried to stop them, stones and bottles came flying at your windows." By the end of the decade, some ten million men would be prematurely dead, mostly from alcohol-related causes and suicide.

In another point for the capitalism-blamers, Russian death rates closely tracked the ups and downs of Russia's GDP. When the economy improved modestly around 1995, mortality fell; when it tanked again in 1998, mortality rose, and the crisis only began to subside with the rise of oil prices and job growth in the mid-2000s. But—in the plus column for the communism-blamers—poverty alone didn't seem to explain what was going on. Women were more affected by unemployment and poverty than men, and yet far more men died from alcohol poisoning and suicide; the alcohol-suicide plague was also concentrated in Moscow, St. Petersburg, and other large cities, rather than in the much poorer countryside. And if boredom and poverty were the sole causes of the alcohol-suicide plague, why did Boris Yeltsin, who was neither bored nor poor, nearly succumb to it too?

Capitalism isn't just a system for moving money and goods around. It's also a culture, a way of life, with its own values and patterns of thought and emotion, that shape our relationships and how we see ourselves. Long before Lenin arrived at Finland Station in 1917 to launch the Soviet era, it had always been an alien system in Russia. Prerevolutionary millionaires built churches to atone for the sin of their avarice, and folk healers refused money, so as not to profit from others' misfortunes.

Under Soviet communism, the inefficient economy forced people to depend on each other for favors, side deals, sharing,

and exchange. Russians call it *Blat*—a system of interdependence
based on it's-not-what-you-know-but-who-you-know petty
corruption that enabled people to access consumer goods and
services that the state was unable to distribute efficiently. In this
way, for all its flaws—and there were plenty—the Soviet Union
created an ethos of cooperation and mutual aid, not under the
dreamworld umbrella of socialist brotherhood, but because few
could survive without cooperation and sharing. Generosity, even
if it only meant alerting someone that someone else was selling
cheap cucumbers somewhere, was the real currency of exchange.

Anthropologist Dale Pesmen lived in the Siberian city of
Omsk during the early 1990s, and documented her Russian
friends' reactions to Yeltsin's economic reforms. To them, there
had always been something obscene about cash. People would
back off and gasp at the sight of it. It was impossible, a friend
told Pesmen, to say "Pay me," even when people needed and
expected compensation. Another informant confided that she
could never tell Russian friends that her mother was a sales-
woman because only bad people sold things for money. Selling
your own potatoes or milk in the market might be okay, but
buying commodities somewhere else in order to sell them at a
higher price to your own people was profiteering.

Watching a televised marathon, Pesmen was struck when
the announcer actually apologized for running commercials
from the event sponsors. When an American producer suggested that a Russian version of *Sesame Street* include a segment with children selling lemonade on the street, the Russian
scriptwriters were appalled.

What mattered far more than money, according to Pesmen,
was what Russians call soul—which they see not as Descartes's

64   mysterious bodily organ, but as something shared, a product of recognition and communion. Beneath the cruel absurdity of the Soviet system existed a substructure of friendships, shared confidences, and long afternoons and evenings drinking in the kitchen. These ties were your social security, your identity, and your bank. When you wanted something, writes political scientist Alena Ledeneva, it was better to get it through a friend. Ordinary Soviets were always giving each other things: "a bushel of oranges in season, a good word for someone's child seeking admission to a particular school; a jump in the line for tickets to a Crimean spa; medicine for a relative; a seat on the Trans-Siberian; high-quality clothes; spare parts for the television set and car; a new electric stove; exemption from compulsory kolkhoz work or presence at a party meeting; caviar when there was no caviar in the shops," and so on. While some might call this petty corruption, it wasn't material enrichment people were after; it was enlargement of one's sphere of relationships. These informal exchanges were never quantified, not because Russians lack a head for figures, but because leaving things amorphous and flexible humanized relationships. The gifts you gave others embedded you in a web of solidarity and communion that had formed the basis for Russian social life for as long as anyone could remember. The shambolic Soviet economy would probably never have survived as long as it did without it.

Capitalism, by contrast, boiled nearly every relationship down to a cold transaction, in which goods are valued precisely to the kopeck. *Secondhand Time*, literary historian Svetlana Alexievich's searing 2013 exploration of the post-Soviet experience, describes how this system descended like an "atom bomb" on the Russian people. Her interlocutors grumbled about how the Soviet ideals of community and equality had been sold out for a bunch of hamburgers, VCRs, pantyhose, and blue jeans. "What is our national idea now, besides salami?" lamented a former low-level Communist Party official.

Some seemed to find the new system positively satanic. Previously, there'd been nothing shameful about being poor. "You [felt] for others . . ." said the official. Nowadays, it was always, "'You're broke? Go to Hell!'"; or "'Kick the weak in the eyes! . . . The streets were filled with these bruisers in tracksuits," she went on. "Wolves! They came after everyone."

"Wild, inexplicable avarice took hold," said another of Alexievich's informants. "The smell of money filled the air."

Old shopping avenues, once home to workers cafeterias, shabby little stores, and places where you could buy bus tickets, were transformed overnight into avenues of casinos, gaudy hotels, banks, designer boutiques, and tourist cafés. The street used to be "for everyone," an older woman told anthropologist Michelle Parsons. Now it was only for "a certain type of people. . . . They won't even let me in there. They will say, 'Grandma, where do you think you are going?'"

On TV, reporters chronicled fistfights breaking out in butcher shops, rats nibbling on corpses in the city morgue, and criminals robbing old people in nursing homes. A Russian friend told anthropologist Nancy Ries that the new Russia was an anti-Disneyland, where "everything was going wrong: a gargantuan theme park of inconvenience, disintegration, and chaos." The phrases "complete ruin" and "total disaster" seemed to echo through every conversation. "How bad can it get?" people wondered.

66   "We're extraterrestrials," a young man explained to Pesmen, "abandoned in a hostile world."

What hurt the Russians she met most, writes Parsons in her insightful monograph *Dying Unneeded: The Social Context of the Russian Mortality Crisis*, weren't the shortages of material goods, the sky-high prices, or even the gun battles, but the feeling that others no longer had a use for them. In conversation after conversation, her informants spoke about not being able to offer anything to others, especially their families. Under the Blat economy of gifts and favors, even the poorest had something to contribute: light bulbs pilfered from the factory where they worked, or berries gathered in the forest. Now, anyone could get light bulbs and berries. What mattered was money, which in the 1990s, all seemed to be in the hands of criminals. Everyone else—meaning the good people—was *Nikdo na Nezhda*—needed by no one.

"I feel sorry for my parents," a Russian woman tells Alexievich, "because they were told flat out that they were pathetic *sovoks* [unreformed Soviets] whose lives had been wasted for less than a sniff of tobacco, that everything was their fault, beginning with Noah's ark, and that now no one needed them anymore . . . their world was shattered. They still haven't recovered."

Swept away with the old sharing economy went the whole idea of friendship, now replaced with the frantic scramble for money. "Before, it had seemed like we didn't need money at all," another woman explained to Alexievich. "In reality, none of us lived in the USSR. . . . We lived in our kitchens . . . you'd go to somebody's house, drink wine, listen to songs, talk about poetry. There's an open tin can, slices of black bread . . . there were common symbols by which we recognized one another. We had our own fashions, our own jokes. Those secret kitchen societies are long gone. And gone with them is our friendship, which we had thought was eternal. . . . There was nothing holier than friendship. That amazing glue was holding everything together."

"Everyone's so eager to talk these days, but no one listens to one another," a former soldier told Alexievich. "We're all living in separate countries [now], even though they're all Russia."

Alexievich was struck by how many stories she heard about suicide. Some of those who took their own lives had fought in World War II. They'd slept rough in the frost and wind and watched comrades fall one by one. One had been a boy when the Germans occupied his village, creating, literally, a river of corpses. Two Jewish boys he knew were torn to shreds by German dogs and his own father disappeared forever. After the war, survivors of German occupation like him were stigmatized as collaborators, but he endured this, too, only to set himself on fire in his back garden during the early 1990s.

Alexievich records and curates what people tell her, but doesn't editorialize. Some of her interlocutors knew people who'd died by suicide, but could only speculate about why they did it. Even those who said they themselves had attempted suicide mostly talked around it, as if searching for something. As they told the stories of their lives, they sometimes stumbled upon long-buried memories, and tears streamed down their faces. It's as though Alexievich were recording the eruption of an emotional volcano.

In 2015, Alexievich won the Nobel Prize for Literature. In an interview with journalist Masha Gessen, she said she was working on two new books on the post-Soviet experience, one about death and old age and the other about love. But when she started

68   interviewing people, she encountered a problem. People who'd come of age under the Soviets didn't know how to speak about their own feelings. "You start talking to them about love, and they talk about how they built Minsk. You start talking to them about old age, and they tell you how difficult life was after the war. It's like they never had a life of their own."

The Soviet system forced people to enact a kind of grace under pressure, a shared stoicism, the subversive intimacy of the prison. In a way, all cultures are prisons—some are just higher security than others. They are where we find our friends, our loves, our work, our sense of right and wrong, our reasons to keep going. The formal and informal rituals of collective societies, like Russia's before the transition, enable people to more easily bury their emotions and endure painful experiences. Capitalism exposes our wounds to the naked air, forcing us to find our own meaning in disappointment, sorrow, joy, and fear. In Western societies, we're so used to that vertiginous, vaguely sickening feeling of loneliness and insecurity that many of us don't even recognize it for what it is. But it's what keeps us awake at night wondering who we are, where we belong, whether we made this or that mistake.

Yeltsin saw himself as Russia's first truly human head of state. The czars had ruled by virtue of their magical, otherworldly inheritance; the Soviets by virtue of the providential mystique of the classless utopian future. But Yeltsin was just a man. All he had was the borrowed ideology of Western-style liberalization, which seemed, at least in the early 1990s, to be bringing Russia to ruin.

Russians warmed to him anyway. Crowds that had just been murmuring to reporters about how frustrated they were with his government were beguiled when he showed up. It was not because of what he said—his speeches tended to be uninspiring—but because of who he was: He seemed to feel their pain, as if he were one of them.

And he did feel it. At night, memories of his university days would come back to him. He'd lived in a tiny communal apartment—what Soviets referred to as "barracks"—with a handful of friends who shared everything. The Soviet Union had few good sides, but for a certain type of young person in the early 1950s, with the war over, living conditions improving slightly, and Stalin soon to be dead, there were real possibilities for bliss. "We lived in an atmosphere of pure friendship," recalls Yeltsin in his memoir *The Struggle for Russia*,

> of a happy and slightly frantic romanticism that now seems simply impossible to imagine. I don't recall ever seeing such fantastic energy ever again—and all against the backdrop of the half-starving, almost ascetic barracks existence of the Soviet Union in those days. The object of our romanticism and emotions were global issues—outer space, communism, the virgin territories. . . . It was all something incredible and immense.

After his second suicide attempt in the spring of 1993, Yeltsin rallied. He managed to squeak through the impeachment vote, and a public referendum on his presidency also went relatively well. In August, he spent time with his family and played tennis. But another ordeal loomed. His former vice president and other hard-line communists were stockpiling machine guns and rocket launchers in the Parliament building; armed

70   gangs allied with them roamed the city, calling once again for Yeltsin to be deposed, this time by force.

Yeltsin had grown up in the foothills of the Ural Mountains, a tough, pioneer region whose people had never been subject to serfdom. As a child, he'd lost his thumb and index finger playing with a grenade; he'd seen his father arrested and sent to one of Stalin's gulags; he'd been stranded in the snow, thrown from a runaway horse cart, and almost crushed by a derailed train. In 1987, he'd resigned from the Politburo. In 1991, he'd fought back against revanchist Soviets by standing on a tank that had been ordered to retake the country. If internal demons were a problem for him, external enemies he could deal with.

At first, the army refused to get involved in the standoff between the Kremlin and the Parliament. It was harvest season and the soldiers, themselves hungry and underpaid, were out gathering potatoes. Finally, Yeltsin ordered them to attack the Parliament, and in October an array of tanks lined up in front of the building and fired rockets at the largely unoccupied upper floors. Images of the assault, broadcast around the world by CNN, showed shards of masonry flying and thousands of pages of documents fluttering out the windows. Nearly two hundred people were killed in the mayhem.

Things finally settled down a bit in 1994, and at that point Yeltsin embarked on a two-and-a-half-year drinking binge that became legendary in diplomatic circles. Previously known to knock back a few tumblers now and then, he now went everywhere with two briefcases: one containing a coded communication system for setting off Russia's nuclear warheads, and another containing two bottles of vodka and a jar of pickled cucumbers. While reviewing departing Russian troops with

Chancellor Helmut Kohl in Berlin, he grabbed the baton from the conductor of a military band and led the musicians in a tipsy rendition of the Russian folk song "Kalinka." A month later, too drunk to get off the plane, he had to cancel a meeting with the Irish prime minister. On a state visit to Washington, DC, in 1995, secret service agents found him wandering around Pennsylvania Avenue at night in his underwear.

By the time Yeltsin had stepped down from the presidency in 1999, he'd been hospitalized for five heart attacks, an ulcer, and multiple cases of double pneumonia, all common among severe alcoholics. He spent so much time in the hospital being watched over by doctors, nurses, aides, and family members that he began, he wrote, to feel like the elephant in the Moscow Zoo, for whom he developed a new sympathy. And yet had he not been cared for in this way, he almost certainly would have died in office, along with millions of other Russians of his generation who'd been traumatized by the collapse of the Soviet Union.

To drink yourself to death, you need to consume about twenty-five shots of vodka, or more than a bottle, all at once. A large man who'd developed some tolerance would have to drink considerably more. Why would millions of Russian men do that? Why would Yeltsin come close to doing it? Perhaps, Dale Pesmen suggests, he and the others were trying to revive that lost feeling of connection and community, without which life felt meaningless.

A paradoxical finding of the many studies of alcoholism in Russia during the 1990s was that the more people drank, the better they said they felt—even as their drinking was killing them. The epidemiologists couldn't explain it, but in her evocative study of the transition years, Pesmen suggests that

72 alcohol served for many Russians as the material essence of the soul: It brought people back together, or seemed to, if only for a while, helping them feel more human as the world hardened around them. A round of drinks blurred the edges of the brutal post-Soviet world, made debt collectors "forget why they came," and muddied the waters of business transactions, leaving behind a warm memory, not a cold, hard deal. Drunken friends blended into each other, sharing memories, stories, gifts. Sometimes a glass of vodka even performed miracles, enabling friends to part with things that seemed to come from nowhere. As a Russian woman tells Alexievich, time spent drinking with friends doesn't count toward your lifespan.

On December 31, 1999, Yeltsin sat, stiff and bloated, before TV cameras and announced that he was stepping down from the presidency. He also apologized to the Russian people. "What we thought would be easy turned out to be painfully difficult," he admitted. "I ask you to forgive me for not fulfilling some hopes of those people who believed that we could jump from the gray, stagnating totalitarian past into the bright, rich, and civilized future in one go . . . it could not be done in one fell swoop." Members of the camera crew cried as he spoke, as did many others during the broadcast later that day.

By then, most Russians were fed up with their country's economic experiments. Nearly 60 percent said on surveys they wanted to return to Soviet times, and roughly one in four said they missed Joseph Stalin. Nostalgia may connote homesickness for the past, or the loss of a dream that never conformed to reality. Alexievich found that even gulag survivors felt it. "What's out there?" said one. "The power of mammon!

No values are left except for the power of the purse." Her son,
a former military officer now trading in Italian plumbing fix-
tures, liked to get drunk with his old army buddies. "By morning, we're putting our arms around each other . . . belting out
Komsomol [Soviet Youth League] songs at the top of our lungs."

On the one hand, he admitted it was sadness; his children
were studying accounting and made fun of Solzhenitsyn. He
worried that, before long, he'd have nothing in common with
them. "But on the other hand," he said, "it was fear."

But of what? He doesn't explain, and Alexievich doesn't
press it. But it's worth noting that among the many political
parties that emerged at that time was the National Bolshevik
Party, whose central principle was the "negation of the individual and his centrality." In the early 2000s, it became the Eurasia
Party, which stressed "obedience and love for one's leader" over
Western "individualism and the independence of opinion." As
of this writing, Vladimir Putin has been ruling Russia, with
the apparent approval of the majority of his people, for a quar-
ter century. It's probably no coincidence that Russia has seen
increasing anti-Semitism in recent years, directed against that
eternally stigmatized symbol of the ruthless creditor who
wants every kopeck of his money back, no matter what.

Yeltsin lived for another seven years. He read voraciously,
entertained visiting dignitaries, and enjoyed the company of his
family, about whom he writes warmly in all three of his mem-
oirs. He also liked riding around in a golf cart. Sometimes, to
his bodyguards' alarm, he'd hare downhill, heading straight for a
tree, swerving just at the last minute to avoid a crash.

Deaths of Despair in America's Heartland

In 2015, newly appointed surgeon general Vivek Murthy set out on a listening tour to find out more about what was ailing Americans. He heard hundreds of stories from people struggling with heart disease, Alzheimer's, cancer, and the cost of health care, but these problems were evident from government statistics; he needn't have left his office to find them. What he would not otherwise have been able to detect otherwise was how lonely Americans were. Countless people spoke to him of shouldering life's burdens alone and feeling their lives meant nothing to anyone. Some patients lay in their hospital beds for weeks without visitors. According to the American Enterprise Institute, the fraction of men who say they have six or more close friends has halved since 1990, and a 2018 Kaiser Family Foundation survey found that 22 percent of adults—fifty-seven million people—said they felt lonely most of the time.

We are wired for connection, Murthy explains in his 2020 book *Together: The Healing Power of Human Connection in a Sometimes Lonely World*. The parts of our brains used for social interaction are firing even when we're alone, like a car idling in the driveway. If we spend too much time alone, the faculty for connection begins to break down. We become distrustful and paranoid, scanning the landscape for threats. The guy who bumps into us on the street or cuts us off in traffic did it on purpose; the boss who didn't acknowledge our greeting in the hall wasn't preoccupied or nearsighted. He hates us. Soon even those who might have been friends are turned off, leaving us lonelier still.

America wasn't always a lonely nation, but for decades, our social life has been withering away. We now spend twenty hours less each month socializing, and twenty-four hours more alone each month than we did in 2003. Since the 1960s, membership in Parent Teacher Associations, bridge clubs, local charities, church groups, arts and crafts groups, veterans' organizations, bowling leagues, and myriad other local associations that once formed the bedrock of American community life has plummeted. Younger people are far less likely to attend picnics, card games, and dinner parties than their parents and grandparents were, and they are also far less likely to read newspapers and participate in town meetings, so they have less to talk about when they do socialize. On surveys, young people are also more likely to say they don't trust their neighbors and that they themselves recently engaged in antisocial behavior, such as speeding through a red light or giving the finger to another driver.

Far more Americans are also making the ultimate decision to disengage. By the 1990s, American adolescents and young adults were three to four times more likely to die by suicide than their 1950s counterparts. The working class—the 70 percent or so of American adults without a four-year college degree—are

76   particularly vulnerable. In the years just after World War II, suicide rates were similar among all social classes. By the mid-2000s, the suicide rate for middle-aged people with bachelor's degrees had barely budged; for those without one, it had quadrupled. The greatest increases were seen in those states and counties where measures of what sociologists call social capital, the density of community organizations and norms of trust and sharing, has declined most steeply—in other words, in those places where people seem to be most lonely.

Not everyone agrees about what is causing our social fabric to fray. In his 2000 book *Bowling Alone: The Collapse and Revival of American Community*, Harvard social capital expert Robert Putnam tentatively pinned the blame on television, which arrived in American homes at peak sociability in the mid-1960s. Rather than going out to meet people at the bowling alley or church supper, Americans could now stay home and watch other people do these things. But Putnam admits that his own statistical analyses suggest TV explains only a small fraction of America's social disconnection. The entry of women into the workforce and suburban sprawl don't explain it either.

Former surgeon general Murthy also takes aim at technology, especially the computers and smartphones that promise to connect us, but leave far too many Americans alone, worrying about how many likes they have. Many troubled young people, especially those whose lives are already overshadowed by family conflict, bullying, substance abuse, and mental illness, may be drawn away from the sustaining relationships they desperately need into dark corners of the internet where people discuss suicide, including methods, with tragic results.

But social media can't explain the longer-term US suicide increase, which began in the 1970s, long before personal computers, let alone smartphones, even existed. Moreover, youth suicides have fallen across Western Europe in the past two decades, even as social media became a sensation there too. There are also controversies about the data linking social media to suicide. The definitions of depression and suicidality used in standard questionnaires were expanded right around the time social media use began to soar, which would tend to increase the number of people deemed to suffer from these conditions, even if there had been no real change.

Social media no doubt plays some role in America's mental health and suicide crisis, but an even greater culprit is the economy itself, which, beginning in the 1970s, switched from emphasizing the welfare of workers to prioritizing the welfare of consumers, investment bankers, and corporate shareholders. This created a vast precariat class beset with family dysfunction and despair.

In 1976, Peter Drucker, the father of corporate management consulting, declared that America had become the first socialist country. Back then, large corporations more or less guaranteed working-class people lifetime employment at good wages, and they also provided health insurance and pensions. It was a better deal, Drucker proclaimed, than Karl Marx or Rosa Luxemburg ever dreamed of.* This hadn't happened by chance. The Great Depression and World War II had obliterated many of America's great fortunes, reducing both inequality and the concentration

---

*Peter Drucker, *The Unseen Revolution: How Pension Fund Socialism Came to America* (HarperCollins, 1976), referred to in Nicholas Lemann, *Transaction Man.*

78   of political power. This, along with a century-long surge in union organizing, fostered a culture of postwar egalitarianism and respect for ordinary workers.* But that social compact was already collapsing, even as Drucker wrote those words.

In the early 1970s, bankers and investors, hit by inflation and the oil crisis, rediscovered an old way to make money: crushing their workforces. They began by farming out tasks like cleaning, security, and so on to independent contractors who cut wages and benefits and subjected workers to overtime theft, exposure to toxic chemicals, and other abuses.† Solidarity had always been labor's great weapon, but this deliberate fissuring of the workplace—as economist David Weil calls it—into myriad subsidiaries meant that to exert significant pressure on an employer now required multiple separate strikes instead of just one. The 1952 Taft–Hartley Act had already imposed restrictions on union activity that made organizing even harder: It forbade workers in one union from striking in sympathy with others, for example, or pressuring their employers not to do business with companies involved in labor disputes, or refusing to handle hot cargo—goods produced by such companies.

Meanwhile, economists at the University of Chicago and their disciples were turning CEOs on to downsizing, offshoring, and monopoly formation, as Washington began permitting banks to engage in takeovers, mergers, and leveraged buyouts and to create complex financial instruments that were neither regulated nor properly understood by most people. From 1997 to 2020

---

* Robert Kuttner, "Why Work Is More and More Debased," *New York Review of Books*, October 23, 2014. See also Thomas Piketty, *Capital in the Twenty-First Century* (Belknap Press, 2014).

† David Weil, *The Fissured Workplace* (Harvard University Press, 2014).

alone, more than ninety thousand factories closed, along with
countless small businesses that served their workers. Millions
of well-paying working-class jobs were lost, and much of the
nation's social capital went with them. Meanwhile, a small number of behemoth corporations transformed the once-variegated
economic landscape of America's towns and smaller cities into
wastelands of highways, box stores, and parking lots.

The economists had done the math. They predicted, cor-
rectly, that moving industries overseas and replacing local firms
with national and multinational behemoths like Walmart and,
eventually, Amazon wouldn't have much effect on the overall unemployment rate; people could still work for the behemoths, and they could always move somewhere else or retrain.
But the economists underestimated the effect of these policies
on two things, the first being working-class wages. The people of
Milwaukee, Wisconsin, for example, went from having the country's second highest median income in 1969 to having the second highest poverty rate among large American cities in 2021,
according to the *New York Times*.

Even worse were the effects on entities economists seldom
measure: the sense of community and the integrity of America's
fragile social ecosystem.* Urban studies professor Charles
Heying was a graduate student in the early 1990s when he, like
Robert Putnam, became interested in the disappearance of
America's voluntary associations. He found that they tended to
be run by the local crème de la crème—businesspeople, news-
paper editors, bankers, politicians, union leaders, and the heads
of local utilities and their spouses, who gave money to the local

* Stephen Marglin, *The Dismal Science: How Thinking Like an Economist
Undermines Community* (Harvard University Press, 2008).

80   concert hall, sponsored church picnics, attended Little League games, and spoke at the Elks Club, where they hobnobbed with potential customers, voters, and—for the editors—sources for local news stories. Ordinary people wanted to hobnob with the elites in return, because they could make things happen—raise money for a new school gym, for example, or change a zoning rule. In other words, it isn't just gardening, softball, and tuna casserole that leads people to join groups and socialize. It's other people with whom they share community concerns.

The power of these local elites collapsed as their businesses were wiped out or taken over by national chains like Walmart, UPS, McDonald's, and Bank of America, with headquarters hundreds or even thousands of miles away. The directors and managers who ran the new chains seldom had local connections and had little interest in engaging in local social life or supporting civic associations. Many expected to move on in a few years anyway.

These companies not only paid workers a tiny fraction of what the firms they displaced had, but they also squelched what was left of the local economy by putting thousands of small merchants out of business through underselling and other dubiously legal anticompetitive tactics. In the wake of deindustrialization, many states, desperate for employers of any kind, gave the new behemoths generous incentives so that some paid little to no local taxes, even though they were served by sanitation, fire, and police departments that now-shuttered local factories, grocery stores, clothing boutiques, and other small businesses once paid for. Hence the many potholes, overgrown and unmaintained parks, homeless encampments, and overburdened local services in many parts of the country that belied the good news about the stock market, unemployment, and inflation.

But the corporate behemoths' greatest casualty may well be the nation's soul. During the 1990s, the Dow rose 430 percent,* even as the Welfare Reform Act pushed millions of poor people into the unskilled labor market, where jobs typically paid a barely survivable $7 an hour.

In 1998, journalist Barbara Ehrenreich decided to apply for a job at Walmart. What makes *Nickel and Dimed*, the book she eventually wrote about her experiences at a series of low-wage jobs, so heroic is that it captures not just the material miseries of poverty—the constant aching feet and joints, the squalor of living in a van or crowded trailer, the inability to afford filling for a sandwich or a stained T-shirt from Walmart's clearance bin— but the struggle against constant humiliation. Stony-faced managers test her urine, search her purse, and warn her that casual chats with colleagues—the one thing that makes boring jobs bearable—are considered "time theft" from the company. "We're nothing to these people," a coworker at a maid service tells Ehrenreich.

Reading Ehrenreich's book, I thought of Katherine Newman's prescient 1988 study of downsizing, *Falling from Grace*, in which older people recalled Elizabeth, New Jersey— where 15 percent of residents now live in poverty—as a "place of grandeur, where ladies and gentlemen in fine dress promenaded down the main avenue on Sunday." There, the Singer Sewing Machine company employed over ten thousand workers, roughly a tenth of the city's population. The company awarded scholarships to children, sponsored baseball games, and hosted dances and bar mitzvahs in its recreation hall. Each

---

* Shep Perkins, "Revisit the '90s playbook for clues to 2025 and beyond," Putnam Investments, November 19, 2024.

82   sewing machine had a label, and if returned with a defect, the man who'd made it would fix it himself.

Walmart, by contrast, treated workers as if they were the ones on the assembly line. To apply for a job there, Ehrenreich had to answer a questionnaire designed to weed out potential troublemakers. Among other questions, she's asked whether she's prone to self-pity, whether she ever thinks people are talking about her behind her back, and whether she thinks nonconformist behavior is ever appropriate. "You will have no secrets from us," Walmart seems to be telling her. "We want your innermost self."

At a diner where Ehrenreich also works briefly, she sneaks free pie and milk to hard-luck customers and puts extra sour cream on their baked potatoes, as a way, she realizes later, of expressing her beleaguered humanity. She stokes feminist solidarity with her coworkers, and marvels at the agility of a more seasoned colleague, who seems to be able to disappear at one end of the restaurant and reappear at the other, like a fairy.

But Ehrenreich can't escape a toxic surge of bitterness, borne of the daily onslaught of indignities, to which she was all but immune in her ordinary life as a writer. At night, she lies awake ruminating about whether a coworker is plotting against her, and punishes herself for screwing up the vacuuming at the maid job. "Slights loom large," she writes, "and a reprimand can reverberate into the night." Pushing a cart of women's wear around Walmart, Ehrenreich thinks of Sisyphus.

Journalist Emily Guendelsberger's 2019 exposé *On the Clock: What Low-Wage Work Did to Me and How It Drives America Insane* brings Ehrenreich's findings up to date. In an Amazon warehouse, Guendelsberger is on her feet for eleven hours a day, her every move tracked electronically by a scanner gun. If she's two minutes late or spends too much time in the bathroom, her paycheck is adjusted accordingly. At an AT&T call center, customers whose complicated billing and connection problems can't immediately be solved become so angry, she fears they'd kill her if they were to ever meet face-to-face. At McDonald's, she's punished for snapping at a customer who's just thrown salad dressing at her.

Guendelsberger estimates, based on an Oxford University study, that roughly half of all American workers have low-paying "on the clock jobs" with virtually no opportunity for creativity or decision-making. A 2022 study of three million workers in Sweden found that having such a job raises the risk of suicide by nearly 50 percent. A similar study in Japan found that it raises a worker's suicide risk fourfold.

White American men—the demographic group most affected by America's post-1970s suicide surge—tend to find their sense of self-respect and community through work, rather than kinship or class solidarity, so their sense of personal worthlessness can be profound when jobs are unstable, humiliating, and/or pay too little to support a dignified existence. In the old days, factory work was dangerous and dirty; thousands died in accidents or succumbed to black lung disease; miners depended on company stores and homes, and those who lost their jobs faced destitution; but they nevertheless felt a sense of solidarity. Most marriages lasted a lifetime, and communities were held together by social clubs, churches, unions, and friendships.

By contrast, the personal lives of today's low-wage workers mirror the instability of their jobs. The vast majority of women with a college degree have all their children in marriage, but most

84   women without one have at least some, if not all, of their children out of wedlock, often with different men. American children experience more changes in stepfathers, stepmothers, and
residences than children in any other wealthy country; according to sociologist Andrew Cherlin, American families may be
the most unstable in the world. This no doubt contributes to
many child development problems that are also common in the
US, including difficulties sitting still and paying attention in
school, disobedience, and destructive behavior. Children with
these issues often find it difficult to enter, let alone finish, college, perpetuating an intergenerational cycle of thwarted potential, which may also be contributing, along with social media, to
a rise in child and adolescent suicides.[*]

Some conservatives, such as the American Enterprise
Institute's Charles Murray and Vice President J. D. Vance, attribute the upheavals of the American family to moral decline. If
only poor people would embrace religion, adopt the family values of their better-educated peers, stop blaming the government, and work harder, they'd be fine, those conservatives say.
But as economists Anne Case and Angus Deaton point out, if
it were really true that workers were slacking off, wages would
have risen for those who weren't; but this hasn't happened.
About half of those who patronize America's food banks live in
households with a working adult—perhaps an Amazon warehouse worker, Uber driver, Walmart greeter, or caregiver—who

[*]C. K. Ormiston, W. R. Lawrence, S. Sulley et al., "Trends in Adolescent
Suicide by Method in the US, 1999–2020," *JAMA Network Open* 7, no. 3
(2024): e244427; Jean M. Twenge, "Increases in Depression, Self-Harm, and
Suicide Among U.S. Adolescents After 2012 and Links to Technology Use:
Possible Mechanisms," *Psychiatric Research and Clinical Practice* 2, no. 1.

doesn't earn enough for groceries. Around 30 percent of homeless adults have jobs.

The French sociologist Pierre Bourdieu was among the first
to characterize the psychological vulnerability of the new intermittently employed, low-wage precariat class. When workers
are made to feel replaceable and lucky to have even a lousy job,
they become cynical, depressed, and easier to exploit. The philosopher Simone Weil, who spent time doing repetitive factory
work in the 1930s, likened it to the feeling of being colonized.
"Nothing in the world," she wrote, "can make up for the loss of
joy in one's work."

Many poor Americans simply turn inward, focusing on
their own personal struggles with trauma and pain. One of
Case and Deaton's most striking findings is what I'll call the
"pain paradox." On national health surveys, sixty-year-old
white Americans without a four-year college degree are
two-and-a-half times more likely to report that their health
is fair or poor than same-aged whites with a BA. Even though
working-class jobs involve less risk and physical exertion than
in the past, each generation of non-BA whites since the Baby
Boom has reported more pain, at younger ages, than the previous one, so that non-BA whites actually report more pain
at age sixty than at age eighty, whereas the reverse is true for
Blacks, whites with a BA, and populations in nineteen compar-
ison countries.

The pain experienced by working-class whites is so severe
it's keeping many of them from working altogether. In 1993,
4 percent of forty-five- to fifty-four-year-olds without a BA
were out of the workforce for health reasons; today, 11 percent
are. In Virginia's coal region, journalist Beth Macy found that in

one county, 60 percent of men were either unemployed or living on disability payments.

This pain seems to be real. It's not that people are faking it in order to live large on food stamps. But a combination of prescription and recreational drug use, sky-high smoking rates, depression, anxiety, and other emotional problems—which may worsen the actual feeling of pain, according to neuroscientists—along with poor access to good health care, seems to have amplified the effects of work injuries, accidents, and the physical and emotional scars of domestic violence and trauma resulting from military service.

Chronic pain, according to a 2013 *JAMA Psychiatry* study, more than doubles the risk of suicide, and US counties where more people report chronic pain also tend to have the highest suicide rates. The communities Guendelsberger describes are disproportionately affected by opioid addiction, alcoholism, and homelessness that haunt previously vibrant streets, once home to factories, small businesses, sports clubs, and other community associations.

This may sound melodramatic but reading about the demise of the generously pro-worker mid-century American economy and the rise of the bottom-line-obsessed behemoth corporation reminded me of the forced settlement of the Inuit, the rapid modernization of Micronesia, and other, older, colonial tragedies. Companies like Walmart, McDonald's, and Amazon aim not only to extract as much wealth as possible from the communities they occupy, but they may also be guilty of what indigenous rights activists call cultural genocide—the destruction of the traditions, values, and institutions that give a people its identity.

What Is Haunting America's Veterans?

Over seven thousand US service members died in the Iraq and Afghan wars, but more than four times as many have taken their own lives since those conflicts began. Prior to 9/11, the suicide rate for military personnel was lower than that for same-aged civilians, but as the Iraq and Afghan conflicts wore on, military suicides, particularly among young veterans, went through the roof. By 2014, the suicide rate for eighteen- to twenty-four-year-old male vets of the so-called "sandbox wars" had jumped to 124 per 100,000—roughly seven times the civilian rate for men in that age group.

Some post-9/11 veteran suicides have been linked to traumatic brain injuries caused by shock waves from heavy artillery, but these can't explain everything. Brain injury—related suicides usually occur in men in their forties who have been deployed multiple times. The post-9/11 veteran suicide spike was concentrated among much younger service members of both sexes, and combat soldiers account for only 25 percent of all post-9/11 military suicides; those with multiple

88   deployments, only 10 percent. In other words, the causes of the post-9/11 suicide spike were most likely to be found not in the material of the brain, but in the software of the mind.

The war-haunted suicidal veteran is an enduring subject of Western art, from Sophocles's *Ajax* to Virginia Woolf's *Mrs. Dalloway* and J. D. Salinger's "A Perfect Day for Bananafish." And yet, Veterans Administration officials didn't expect that the Iraq and Afghan wars would spark a suicide epidemic on such a scale. While post-traumatic stress—debilitating flashbacks, anxiety, paranoia, hyperreactivity, and anger—is common among veterans of all generations, Vietnam veterans, contrary to popular belief, seem not to have been more likely to die by suicide than civilians, regardless of age, race, ethnicity, combat experience, and other variables. Nor is there evidence of elevated suicides among service members from previous conflicts.

Sophocles, Woolf, and Salinger weren't wrong. It's just that their stories may have been incomplete. In 2020, Yale psychologist Brandon Nichter and colleagues found that veterans who had deployed to combat were at heightened risk of suicide, but this risk was amplified among those who had experienced abuse in childhood, a finding that has been replicated by other researchers. This isn't surprising. Child abuse is one of the strongest known risk factors for suicide. American adults who report having experienced physical, sexual, or emotional abuse as children are two to five times more likely to have attempted suicide at least once, and more severe abuse is associated with greater frequency and seriousness of attempts. Hong Kong adolescents hospitalized after a suicide attempt were found to be four to six times more likely to have experienced sexual or physical abuse than adolescents hospitalized with influenza.

Australian child sexual abuse survivors were found to be ten to thirteen times more likely to die by suicide than other young Australians.

Most people who were abused as children don't become suicidal, and some who weren't, do, but the combination of childhood and adult trauma seems to be particularly damaging to the will to live. One interpretation of Nichter's finding is that part of the mechanism of adult trauma—whether it's witnessing or participating in the horrors of war, being raped, or something else—involves the reexperiencing of painful emotions, particularly feelings associated with betrayal, that echo—consciously or otherwise—through the lives of survivors, making every subsequent trauma that much harder to bear. Even when the wounds of child abuse seem to have scarred over, and even for those whose experiences of childhood trauma were relatively mild, extreme military experiences—and presumably other serious adult traumas—can tear open old wounds so they bleed afresh. It's not that those with abuse-free childhoods don't risk severe mental illness and even suicide when they experience adult trauma; they do. But childhood trauma may amplify that profound loneliness that makes us feel unworthy of existence.

It so happens that the United States has a serious child abuse problem, and many military personnel are affected by it. After 9/11, some two hundred fifty thousand young Americans signed up for military and national guard service, the most rapid recruitment since Pearl Harbor. Most were middle-class kids from rural and suburban towns throughout the country. They were, in many respects, the muscle of the country—brave, physically healthy, and patriotic. But later surveys revealed that they were twice as likely to have been physically and sexually abused

90   as children, and to have witnessed domestic violence, compared to same-aged civilians. In other words, many of them may have joined up not only to defend their country against terrorism, but also to get away from tormentors in their own homes.

For this book, I interviewed over two dozen veterans who'd tried, at one time or another, to take their own lives. Some had been hospitalized after attempts and come close to death. I found them through acquaintances and veteran support groups, and they belonged to all recent military generations— post-9/11 back to Vietnam. None of the vets mentioned brain injuries, suggesting they saw their troubles as psychological, not physiological.

Virtually all the war traumas they described had to do with what military psychologists call moral injury—the long-term psychological impact of witnessing or committing acts that clash with one's own moral views, such as killing civilians, seeing fellow soldiers killed when it could have been them, being betrayed by a more senior officer, being sexually assaulted by a fellow soldier, and other jolts to the sense of trust and community. The modern American military with its leave-none-behind ethos promises a sense of belonging not so different from traditional Micronesia or Nunavut. In boot camp, recruits are bullied and screamed at by officers, but they are also taught solidarity. They are trained to fight not for an ideal or cause—theirs is really not to reason why; the president and the Pentagon do that—but for each other. The goal is to keep your buddies safe and alive and to behave honorably. But both Vietnam and the post-9/11 wars were controversial from the get-go, and their conduct was rife with strategic and tactical blunders that cost countless civilian and military lives. Many of those who witnessed or were involved in them have told journalists, congressional committees, and their friends and relatives that they experienced a sickeningly suicidogenic cocktail of guilt, shame, dread, and deep loneliness as a result.

"There is no way to explain what it's like to take a human life," explains Claude AnShin Thomas, who nearly took his own life after serving as a helicopter door gunner in Vietnam. He eventually became a Buddhist monk and now offers spiritual counseling to other troubled veterans. "To see people around you killed in various ways, I can't get my head around it even now," he told me. Many vets tamp down their emotions with psychiatric medications or recreational drugs, but relief is fleeting. The vets we lose, Thomas says, are those who are so medicated, they end up feeling nothing. "And they look around and go, 'If I don't feel anything. What's the point?'"

When I set out to interview veterans, I expected to—and did—hear harrowing war stories. But I hadn't expected so many harrowing child-abuse stories. The subject usually came up incidentally, when I asked the vets about their backgrounds. Most came from middle-class families with no outward signs of dysfunction. But everyday life for the children sounded utterly terrifying. Some had parents who were alcoholics; some had learning disabilities and were bullied in school in front of everyone, even by teachers; most had witnessed their fathers beating their mothers and had been beaten themselves by fathers, mothers, grandmothers, or older brothers. One told me his violent, alcoholic father forced him, at age eleven, to drown the puppies of his beloved cocker spaniel.

"Ma had a signal when Dad was in a bad mood," said Max (a pseudonym), whose father typically began the day with a shot of

92   spirits. "One finger meant he was okay. Five meant he was about to explode."

Max's father, a Vietnam Navy SEAL vet, had come home with what would later be known as PTSD. One night when Max was three, his father nearly killed the whole family. They were driving home from a party when Dad, drunk as usual, began screaming at Max's mother. Then he blacked out. The vehicle wove into oncoming traffic, horns blared, headlights flooded the cab, and everyone was screaming. Finally, they veered off the road and Max's dad ended up passed out on the grass. He stopped drinking the next day, but his rages continued intermittently until Max was around twelve.

Max did his military service stateside and never saw combat, but this didn't spare him moral injury, which psychologists now recognize does not depend on battle experiences. In his early twenties, he found himself working with a team that managed the nuclear arsenal. Before long, he began to experience nightmares, which he attributed to disgust at working with weapons that could destroy the whole world. He started drinking heavily and taking and selling drugs, which eventually got him kicked out of the military. Then he bounced around taking classes, doing odd jobs, and having troubled relationships with women.

In 2011, a fiancée whom he loved but quarreled with abandoned him. "Where she lived inside me got ripped out," he said, "and all this pain spewed forth." It came not just from the failed relationship, he explained to me, but also from intergenerational war trauma and his own troubled past. Sometimes he'd lie awake at night sobbing. Coworkers waved their hands in front of his face because, as he put it, he just wasn't there. Driving alone at night, he struggled to keep from steering into a tree or off the edge of a cliff. Only prayer and, eventually, psychotherapy kept him from suicide.

Max's story came back to me months later when I learned of a study carried out by the Scottish psychoanalyst Ronald Fairbairn, who treated World War II soldiers suffering from similar symptoms. Back then, it was called shell shock: extreme anxiety, nightmares, insomnia, irritability, guilt, shame, and suicidal thoughts in previously normal men that didn't subside with time away from the battlefield. Fairbairn was struck by how preoccupied these men were, in life and in their dreams, not just with battlefield horrors, but also with childhood ones—abandonment, beatings, humiliation, helplessly watching their fathers beat their mothers.

In Fairbairn's day, most psychoanalysts were strict Freudians, who maintained that adult neuroses resulted from an inability to manage universal innate drives for sex and other forms of gratification, as well as drives for risk-taking and destruction. Fairbairn helped establish Object Relations Theory, the idea—more widely accepted now—that adult mental health problems often stem from abuse, neglect, and other traumas in early childhood that remain unattached to conscious memory, emerging only in dreams and when traumatic events evoke similar feelings.

Fairbairn came up with a theory that helps explain how war experience—and presumably other forms of extreme adult trauma—can cause childhood scars to erupt in terrifying ways. He referred to it as dissociation, a powerful defense mechanism—first intensively studied by French physician and psychologist Pierre Janet—that forces into the unconscious

94   memories too painful for the child's developing personality to deal with. Together, these memories form a sub-personality that, according to the theory, "knows" about events the conscious self cannot accept. This sub-personality is completely cut off from the conscious self and only emerges when triggered by external events such as trauma.* It's as if, Fairbairn wrote, the hated self remained buried in the basement of the mind like an evil spirit, only to reemerge with a vengeance in times of stress.

Fairbairn wasn't the only one who saw this. A 1946 study comparing twenty World War II veterans who'd been discharged with neuropsychiatric problems with controls who'd served out their enlistment terms found the groups didn't differ in their attitudes to the war, combat experience, or even in outward measures of childhood adversities such as parental deaths or broken homes. What distinguished the neuropsychiatric cases from the others was the emotional tone of the families they'd grown up in. The controls said they'd had affectionate relationships with both parents, whom they liked and respected, even when they were strict. The neuropsychiatric patients tended to describe their fathers as cold, indifferent, or cruel; only one of the neuropsychiatric cases said his childhood had been happy. Most had been shy, moody children who were easily hurt; as adults, they tended to embark on impulsive marriages that quickly turned sour, and took the deaths of fellow soldiers particularly hard.

For Fairbairn the worst thing about child abuse is the tendency of adults to deny it. Children learn to handle strong emotions just as they learn to walk and use a fork—with the help

* Immense gratitude to Fairbairn scholar David Celani for clarifying this point.

of, hopefully, tender and sympathetic adults. But when abused children turn to their abusers or others in the family, they are often told that whatever happened wasn't so serious, or even that it didn't happen at all. This, according to Hungarian psychoanalyst Sandor Ferenczi, another early Object Relations pioneer, is what really causes the psyche to crack. The abused child, alone with his feelings and now forced to collude in the family denial, is truly lost.

During the 1930s, Fairbairn ran an orphanage for children who'd been removed from their homes because of abuse. He was amazed that even those who'd been beaten within an inch of their lives nevertheless longed to be reunited with their parents. When Fairbairn asked one such eight-year-old whether she'd like him to find her a new kind of mother, she responded like a little soldier: No. "I want my own Mummy."

Virtually none of the institutionalized children saw their parents as bad; instead, they tended to see themselves as bad. Fairbairn theorized that children are programmed to love their parents no matter what, and desperately try to believe that their love is returned. To think otherwise would mean living in an unbearably lonely and insecure world. But this leaves abused children with little alternative but to see themselves as their parents see them, as bad children unworthy of love. As Fairbairn describes the child's resulting emotional firestorm, it sounds a lot like war, but it's a war against the self, which is the essence of moral injury

I'm no psychoanalyst, but Max's story, and those of many of the other vets I spoke with, conveyed to me how their wartime experiences brought back the battlefields of childhood. When Claude AnShin Thomas was five years old, his mother threw

96   him, along with his bike, down the stairs. Both parents rou-
tinely beat him black and blue. Home from the war, he got married and had a son of his own. But he couldn't stand it when the
baby cried. Instead of helping his wife comfort the child, he'd
sometimes just storm out of the house and get high. When the
boy was three, Claude left for good. He tried therapy and got off
drugs, but then one night in 1983, alone in his apartment, he
downed, he says, a thousand barbiturate tablets. In the hospital, the doctor asked him if he planned to do it again. "Yes," he
replied.

Only years later did Thomas begin to understand his reactions. At a Buddhist retreat in upstate New York, he met the
famous monk Thich Nhat Hanh, who'd been exiled from his
native Vietnam in 1966 for his outspoken opposition to the war.
Thich's kind face evoked a memory, long buried in Thomas's
mind. "At some point, maybe six months into my service in
Vietnam," Thomas writes in his memoir, *At Hell's Gate*,

> we landed outside a village and shut down the engines of
> our helicopters.... Often when we shut down near a village
> the children would rush up and flock around the helicop-
> ter, begging for food, trying to sell us bananas or pineapples
> or Coca-Cola, or attempting to prostitute their mothers or
> sisters. On this particular day, there was a large group of
> children, maybe twenty five.... [O]ften the Vietcong would
> use children as weapons against us. So someone chased
> them off by firing an M60 machine gun over their heads.
> As they ran away, a baby was left lying on the ground, cry-
> ing, maybe two feet from the helicopter in the middle of
> the group. I started to approach the baby along with three

or four other soldiers. . . . That is what my non-war conditioning told me to do. But in this instance, for some reason, something felt wrong to me. And just as the thought began to rise in my head to yell at the others to stop . . . just before that thought could be passed from synapse to speech, one of them reached out and picked up the baby, and it blew up. Perhaps the baby had been a booby-trap, a bomb. Perhaps there had been a grenade attack or a mortar attack at just this moment. Whatever the cause, there was an explosion that killed three soldiers and knocked me down, covering me with blood and body parts.

As that memory resurfaced, Claude realized that he'd left his son and the boy's mother not because he couldn't stand to be with them, but because his extreme moral injury had left him unable to stand being in his own skin.

When George (a pseudonym), who'd been a helicopter crew member during the Vietnam War, returned to the States, he nearly lost his mind. Sleepless, paranoid, and angry, he was so easily triggered into rages that he frightened his own psychiatrist. Sometimes he'd stand at the edge of a high bridge, or put a rope around his neck. At night, he dreamed Vietcong and German soldiers were chasing and shooting at him from machine gun nests, as rockets howled around his head. It was even more terrifying, he told me, than what he'd experienced in Vietnam.

"My mother had mood swings," George said casually, later in the interview. "I guess she'd be diagnosed bipolar now. . . . She used to smack us around . . . chasing us, hitting us." Anything could trigger her. His sister had scars no one could explain.

98   Stephan Wolfert grew up in a Midwestern town known for its summer beer and pretzel fests. Unfortunately, it was also known for child abuse, at least among the victims. Many of Stephan's classmates came to school with cuts and bruises. One kid had cigarette burns on his arms. Stephan's own mother beat him frequently, and made it clear that she wished he'd died in the womb. His father, a gentle old drunk, did nothing to stop it. Instead, he'd take the boy to the bar and then ask him not to tell his mother where they'd been. Stephan lied to protect his dad; his mother saw through it, and he got another beating.

When Stephan was five, he "had a thing happen"—as he put it to me—that he couldn't interpret. He was sexually abused, he says—he didn't say by whom—but when he told his mother, she ignored it.

Stephan joined the military in the 1990s and loved it. He even dug basic training. "For two weeks, they called us a piece of shit. I thought, 'Wow, I'm home!' They broke down that piece of shit and turned me into a soldier."

He rose quickly to the rank of lieutenant. Then, during a training exercise in California, rounds from a Bradley Fighting Vehicle hit an armored personnel carrier, killing a close friend. In the months that followed, two of Stephan's subordinates took their own lives—one of whom Stephan had just chewed out for failing to properly secure a vehicle. Consumed with grief and moral injury and in fear for his soul, Stephan went AWOL.

A few years later, he was temping at a catering company in Los Angeles when he found himself at a *Princess Diaries 2* after-party. Tables had been set up in a park across the street from the movie theater, and after the screening hundreds of little kids rushed over for cake and soda, served by actors dressed up as Disney characters.

The scene was total chaos. Four Cinderellas had been fired for losing their tempers in recent weeks. Stephan's job was to clean up fallen blobs of cake, mushed-up napkins, and other children's party detritus. He was squatting over one such mess when he glanced up and found himself eye to eye with a little girl—perhaps five years old. As he recounts in *Cry Havoc!*, his one-man play about enduring military trauma,* she looked him over, laughed, and lobbed a piece of cake in his face. Without thinking, he lunged, arms outstretched, as if to strangle her.

Freaked out but unharmed, the little girl ran screaming to her mother. Stephan dropped everything, rushed back to his apartment, and spent the night with a shotgun in his mouth, hammer back. He removed it only to take an occasional gulp of whiskey. The weird thing was, Stephan told me two decades after the event, the person he saw when he lunged at the little girl wasn't an enemy soldier, or even a nasty drill sergeant. It was his own five-year-old self. And he hated that little kid's guts. It would be years before he finally forgave him.

* *Cry Havoc!* A theater piece by Stephan Wolfert. Available on YouTube, with an introduction by Bessel van der Kolk here: https://www.youtube.com/watch?v=Qr-QI_cGR04.

The Arts of
Endurance

After Stephan Wolfert went AWOL from the military, he wound up somewhere in Montana. In the service, he'd studied history and had had no interest in theater, but one evening, he happened to wander into a performance of Shakespeare's *Richard III* and was gripped by the story of the tyrant king who felt at peace only in battle, and whose mother said she wished she'd strangled him "in her accursed womb."

The play resonated in other ways too. There was something in the cadence of Shakespeare's lines that both calmed and bolstered him, like the rhythmic breathing and marching he'd learned in the army. Eventually, he discovered a love of acting, and went on to establish the dramatherapy nonprofit De-Cruit, which helps troubled veterans reconnect with their own feelings by reciting passages from Shakespeare and drafting and performing theatrical monologues based on their own lives. This is the work that he thinks saved him.

I set out to write about suicide because I felt that if we knew more about why people did it, we might also learn something

about what people live for, and why most people can endure even
the worst hardships without giving up. For some, the causes of
suicidality will always reside in "the internal world, devious,
contradictory, labyrinthine," as the British poet Al Alvarez put
it, and may be entirely neurochemical. But for people swept up
in suicide epidemics, the trials of life seem to be decisive, rais-
ing the question of whether, if some life experiences can ignite
suicidal feelings, perhaps others can help tame them. Most of
the veterans I interviewed for this book were over fifty. They'd
managed to overcome their suicidal feelings and build fairly
happy lives. What, I wondered, did they think had helped them
most?

The answers are important. The Defense Department
has spent billions of dollars on mental health and suicide
prevention—mostly for psychotherapy and antidepressants.
These treatments have helped countless suicidal patients survive, but veteran suicides remain very high, in part because the
Veterans Administration has yet to find a surefire method of
prevention, and also because those services that do exist failed
to meet demand even before the Trump administration began
slashing VA funding—a move that will no doubt cost lives,
although because funds for debt collection have also being cut,
we may never know how many.

In his 2014 book, *The Body Keeps the Score*, psychiatrist
Bessel van der Kolk sheds light on why suicide prevention is
so challenging, especially for veterans. Antidepressant drugs
take the edge off strong emotions, but they can make people
feel weirdly detached, and they sometimes intensify suicidality, especially in young people. Talking cures can be very effective, especially where a strong relationship develops between

102   therapist and patient, but they help only those who can do it. Nearly half of veterans who initiate VA therapy programs drop out, probably because they have difficulty talking about their feelings, and the short duration of many therapies offered by the overstretched VA makes it hard for them to overcome this.

The problem with trauma, as van der Kolk and his psychiatrist colleague Judith Herman maintain, is that it floods the brain with confusing emotions, even as it suppresses the parts of that same organ that help us make sense of our feelings, and enable us to construct a coherent narrative about them. This is why survivors of rape and torture so often freeze up or break down when giving testimony in court.

Because trauma engraves itself on the brain and body, healing from it may require, in addition to therapy, real experiences, in the real world. In *The Body Keeps the Score*, van der Kolk discusses a number of techniques that seem to have helped many of his own patients—including mindfulness, yoga, and neurofeedback techniques that may help people gain control over their heart rate and other normally involuntary processes that correlate with stress. But van der Kolk's last chapter, about the potentially healing effects of theater, music, and other artistic endeavors, interested me most, because every one of the formerly suicidal vets I spoke with had, like Stephan, become an artist of some kind. Very few had considered themselves artists before, but perhaps just as meaningless work can kill you, meaningful work, including artistic expression, may help troubled people confront their sorrows and find narrative coherence and a place in the human conversation.

Everett Cox, a vet with whom I had an extended email correspondence, would only answer some of my questions in verse.

Claude AnShin Thomas wrote a memoir about his conver-
sion to Buddhism and a life devoted to compassion and peace.
Former army medic Jenny Pacanowski writes poetry and leads
an arts group called Women Veterans Empowered and Thriving.
Charlie Pacello's play *Orestes on Skid Row* follows the story of a
homeless vet, who, like Aeschylus's eponymous hero, becomes
a "berserker"—who'll slaughter anyone who threatens him.
Andy (a pseudonym), who accidentally killed an entire family in
Afghanistan, makes soapstone carvings of children, giving each
one an Arabic name. Vietnam combat vet Brian Delate became
an actor and playwright. In his one-man show *Guardian Angels*,
a vet suffering from PTSD is kidnapped by aliens and spends a
year on another planet in the arms of an orgasmic she-spirit.

Virtually all of these artistic projects contained a strong
element of advocacy, usually having to do with the moral injuries of war. In December 2023, I attended a public ceremony
sponsored by a veteran support group in Philadelphia. A retired
army chaplain and a psychologist led the men in readings of
anti-war poetry, Buddhist chants, candle lighting, and a healing circle. Some of the vets also gave personal testimonies about
their war experiences. Midway through, an elderly vet spoke
movingly about how his entire adult life had been haunted by
his accidental killing of a Vietnamese civilian. The performance
wasn't smooth—he fumbled with his glasses, went to the
podium at the wrong time, and had to be shown how to use the
microphone. Afterward, I learned that he hadn't participated in
rehearsals or the months-long group psychotherapy part of the
program. The organizer smiled when he told me this, as though
apologizing for the man. But I saw what the old vet was doing.
Like Walt Whitman, who volunteered in a hospital during the

104 Civil War, he wanted to sing a song of himself. "I'm not a therapy case," he seemed to be saying. "I'm here because I want the world to know who I am, and listen to me."

Art has been used to heal the wounds of war for millennia, writes therapist Ed Tick, who's been working with troubled vets since the 1970s and is also the author of numerous books including *War and the Soul*. Ancient Samurai weren't issued weapons until they'd mastered an art form so they'd be able to cope with their emotions when they returned from battle; Native American warriors were quarantined away from the main camp so they could share their war stories with a medicine man before returning to their families; many of the Greek tragedies were written by Peloponnesian War vets, and may have served as a form of communal healing.

Experimental trials have found that writing, drama, and art therapy may reduce PTSD symptoms in veterans and other trauma survivors. How does it work? No one really knows, but people have been making art since the dawn of the human species, and even before. Designs on rocks have been found in two-hundred-thousand-year-old human settlements. Neanderthals made cave paintings and necklaces, and, according to anthropologists, a three-million-year-old Australopithecine who walked on two legs but looked otherwise much like a gorilla, may have carried around the oldest object on Earth that was treated like a piece of art—a pebble that looked like a face.

Art touches something inside us that philosophers and scientists have been struggling to define for centuries. I suspect it has something to do with recognition, or what psychoanalysts call intersubjectivity, the experience of feeling with others—the feeling that your feelings are respected—the thing so many suicidal people say they don't feel.

At the end of his life, Russian novelist Leo Tolstoy was a curmudgeon. He decided he hated the music of Bach and Wagner and the poetry of Beaudelaire and even deemed some of his own books to be failures. But the theory at the heart of his brief, cantankerous 1897 polemic "What Is Art?" goes some way in explaining the relationship between art and suicide.

Tolstoy had been moved by the way his wife, Sonia, took comfort in music after the death of one of their sons. He theorized that art is successful when the artist reaches to the depths of his soul, pulls out something raw and emotional, and then transforms it so the rest of us feel it too.

Spanish poet Federico García Lorca called it *duende*, meaning "elf." The mystical enchantment of art, he wrote, lies not in technical perfection, but in the artist's ability to convey a pure and reckless cry from the depth of the soul, an assertion of self in the face of despair, as if the artist would die if he didn't express himself, and might die anyway. "With duende, there is neither map nor discipline," Lorca wrote.

> We only know it burns the blood like powdered glass, that it exhausts, rejects all the sweet geometry we understand. . . . The *duende* won't appear if [the artist] can't see the possibility of death, if he doesn't know he can haunt death's house, if he's not certain to shake those branches we all carry, that do not bring, can never bring, consolation.

Making art, or finding meaning in the art of others, can sometimes break the spell of mental isolation, but it's no cure-all for suicidal feelings. As British poet and literary critic Al Alvarez notes, it's probably no coincidence that so many modern artists took their own lives: Artur Rimbaud, Vincent van Gogh, Viginia Woolf, Hart Crane, Joe Orton's boyfriend—who also killed Orton—Caesare Pavese, Paul Celan, Randall Jarrell, Ernest Hemingway, Modigliani, probably Jackson Pollock, and many others.

We understand these artists' work differently, knowing their fates. Sylvia Plath's poems seem to have been squeezed out of her, as if under pressure from the pain and confusion in her heart; Marc Rothko's paintings of numinous boxes within boxes of color can be seen as projections on canvas of the artist's soul as he tries to contain his own inner storms.

Do artists have some special sensitivity to life's slings and arrows? Or is it that modern life can both make us suicidal and inspire a new, yearning form of expression, in which the artist proclaims her inner self to a heartless world through symbols?

Alvarez's quest to understand the relationship between art and suicide was inspired by the death of his friend, the poet Sylvia Plath, in the bitterly cold London winter of 1963. Shortly before taking her own life, Plath visited Alvarez and read him some of her last poems, which would appear posthumously in *Ariel*, the final masterpiece that secured her reputation.

Plath also informed Alvarez that she and her husband, the handsome, brilliant poet Ted Hughes, had split up and she was now looking for a rental.

"I asked no questions," Alvarez writes, "and she offered no explanations." But as she sat cross-legged on his sitting room

floor, the poems poured out of her like some kind of "spirit
possession."

At the time, Hughes was far more famous than Plath, and Alvarez speculates that she was jealous of his literary success. "At a certain pitch of creative intensity," he writes, "it must be more unbearable for the Muse to be unfaithful to you with your partner than for him, or her, to betray you with a whole army of seducers."

But this reader wonders if Alvarez, himself a struggling poet at the time, might not have been projecting. We now know that Hughes had been unfaithful, not just with the two-timing muse, but also with a real woman. No doubt, this hurt Plath, who'd been an astonishing success at nearly everything she put her hand to, and took failure immensely hard. Hughes destroyed Plath's final journals, so we'll never know, but we do know that her last poems deal eloquently with death, violence, suicide, anger, and bad marriages.

Alvarez stiffly praised Plath's craftsmanship and offered some technical suggestions on meter and metaphor. But in the stifling world of Anglo-American postwar conformity, he seems to have been incapable of comforting her. Would Plath have survived had Alvarez been able to listen to her, and not just to her poems? If she'd felt able to cry to him about Hughes's betrayal, over a glass of Scotch? If he'd hugged her and begged her to endure? Perhaps not; but shame and grief magnify in silence, as if in the vacuum of a bell jar.

"A book," Franz Kafka famously wrote, "must be the axe for the frozen sea within us." For whatever reason, Plath's poems failed to break Alvarez's ice. At the end of *Savage God*, Alvarez reveals a likely reason for his reticence. At around the same

108   time, his own marriage was breaking up, and he himself nearly died from an overdose. His problems—a collapsing marriage, professional disappointment—were much the same as Plath's. But she was braver than he was; the effect on the soul of writing such poetry, Alvarez suggests, can be as risky as handling dynamite is to the body.

Suicide, Alvarez concludes, is neither a moral failing nor a disease; it's a "terrible, but utterly natural reaction to the strained, narrow, unnatural necessities" that we "create for ourselves" from modern life's absurdities.

Writing 150 years before Alvarez, Arthur Schopenhauer foresaw that the fundamental subject of nonreligious Western art from his time forward would be just this sort of despair:

> Every epic and dramatic poem can only represent a struggle, an effort, and fight for happiness, never enduring and complete happiness itself. It conducts its heroes through a thousand difficulties and dangers to the goal; as soon as this is reached, it hastens to let the curtain fall; for now there would remain nothing for it to do but to show that the glittering goal in which the hero expected to find happiness had only disappointed him, and that after its attainment he was no better off than before. Because a genuinely enduring happiness is not possible, it cannot be the subject of art.

T. S. Eliot saw poetry as a chemical reaction in which emotions and ideas combine into something totally new under the influence of the catalysis of the poet's mind. As in chemistry, the catalyst itself should remain unchanged in the process. The key to good poetry, as he saw it, was detachment, an "extinction of personality." "Poetry is not a turning loose of emotion," he wrote, "but an escape from emotion; it is not the expression of personality, but an escape from personality. But, of course, only those who have personality and emotions know what it means to want to escape from these things."

For some, escape is not possible. The twentieth century saw a steep increase in the number of writer suicides—so many that it may constitute yet another epidemic.* If so, the explanation may be partly genetic; writers are inordinately prone to bipolar disorder,† and some do their most original work in the throes of mania, before plummeting into despair and self-hatred.‡ But these cycles may have been amplified in recent times by the writer's immersion in the modern battle over identity. Never before has the world been so fractured, never before has it been so easy to feel that whatever you say, and however important you believe it to be, no one will really understand you, and maybe what you're saying is all wrong anyway. In writing this book and other things, I've occasionally glimpsed what my friend the writer Jean Stein may have felt—and perhaps Tolstoy too, near the end of their lives. We are all Ancient Mariners now.

I only came close to suicide once—not just thinking about it, but really planning it, as though it was an obvious thing to do that would solve not only my own problems, but everyone else's

* Mark Seinfelt, *Final Drafts: Suicides of World-Famous Authors* (Prometheus, 1999).

† Simon Kyaga et al., "Mental Illness, Suicide and Creativity: 40-Year Prospective Total Population Study," *Journal of Psychiatric Research*, 47, no.1 (2013): 83–90.

‡ Kay Redfield Jamison, *Touched with Fire: Manic-Depressive Illness and the Artistic Temperament* (Free Press, 1996).

too. A psychologist had recommended Selective Serotonin Reuptake Inhibitors, or SSRIs. Among the most widely prescribed drugs in America, they've helped millions of people with the kind of ruminating low-grade panic and depression I'd spent much of my life experiencing. But they can also intensify suicidal thoughts and behavior, and they did so for me.

The only way I can think of to describe how it felt is to refer readers to Franz Kafka's 1915 masterpiece, *The Metamorphosis*. In the story, salesman Gregor Samsa wakes up to find he's been transformed overnight into a giant bug. His once-doting mother faints when she sees him, and his father chases him away, hissing and stamping his foot until Gregor retreats under the couch. His sister tries at first to be kind, preparing dishes of rotten food, which Gregor, like all bugs, enjoys. But the loneliness gets to him, and he gradually stops eating.

One evening, Gregor hears his sister playing the violin for three young lodgers who are staying with the family. When he was well, Gregor had paid for her violin lessons, bringing art into the family's otherwise dreary life. Now, weak and covered in dust, Gregor is drawn out of his room by the music, which moves him to tears. But upon seeing him, the lodgers declare in disgust that they're leaving, and won't pay their bill.

Now even Gregor's sister has had enough. As he crawls back into his room, she and his parents plot to get rid of him. But he dies that night, thinking of "his family with emotion and love."

Kafka himself died nine years after *The Metamorphosis* appeared, much as Gregor did. He'd had tuberculosis, which he seems to have deliberately accelerated by ignoring his treatment and eating only sporadically. Art doesn't save everyone. Countless artists have taken their own lives. But we'll never know whether they'd have done so sooner if they hadn't at least tried to reach others through their art.

Not everyone is artistically inclined, although many people who think they aren't may not realize that they are. But there is another thing that may help suicidal people. Numerous small studies of psychedelic drugs, such as psilocybin, ayahuasca, ecstasy, and LSD, have found that they can sometimes reduce suicidal thoughts and plans in samples of clinically depressed people, and they may work via mechanisms that are similar to art: by helping people see their problems as part of the human condition, enabling them to communicate more openly, overcome their sense of shame, exclusion, and loneliness, and bond socially with others.

Psychedelic drugs don't work for everyone, and they can have troubling side effects, including suicidality itself, especially in those with severe mental illnesses such as psychosis and bipolar disorder. Research into the mental health effects of psychedelic drugs may also have been subject to biases and the influence of wishful advocates for the drugs, some of whom have even claimed psychedelics have the potential to end war and exploitation and promote world peace. But for some troubled people, the drugs seem to help more than just about anything else.

No one understands how psychedelic drugs work, but according to one model of depression, the parts of the brain that fire when we think about ourselves, and that are theorized to link our feelings and emotions to our sense of self, become ossified into self-defeating negative patterns that are difficult to break without intervention. MRI studies suggest psychedelics make the brain less modular, and its interconnections more

112   random, fluid, and unpredictable. I'm reminded of those public service ads from the 1980s that likened the drug-addled brain to a fried egg. If this model of how psychedelics work is correct, the drugs don't cook the brain; life does. Psychedelics, for some people at least, seem to uncook it, so it can function more flexibly. Electroconvulsive therapy and transcranial magnetic stimulation, which have also helped some suicidal people, may work in similar ways.

This loosening of mental patterns may account for the feeling of egolessness some people who take psychedelic drugs say they experience. As the trip wears off, the brain's connections are hypothesized to reconfigure in more supple ways, enabling a more creative, less rigid sense of self that may be more open to experience and change. In one recent study, depressed people given psychedelics in a therapeutic setting told researchers that the drugs helped them connect with other people, express and understand their own emotions, feel sympathy for themselves, and recognize their struggles as universally human, rather than as uniquely personal and shameful defects.

Psychedelics also seem to increase brain levels of oxytocin, a hormone that promotes pair bonding and intimacy. This may help people suffering from social isolation and depression become less fearful of confiding in others, potentially enabling psychotherapy, the possibility of friendship and community, and that sense of being seen and heard that makes us feel real. Many participants in experimental studies of these drugs have told researchers they went on to make real changes in their lives, traveling, learning new languages, getting new jobs, making long overdue home repairs, taking up rock climbing,

volunteering with refugees, and taking classes, especially in
the performing arts.

The effects of psychedelics fade after a few months or
years, but researchers hope that if the FDA eventually approves
them, they could make psychotherapy more effective for those,
including many troubled veterans, who otherwise seem unable
to benefit from it. The point is not for them to become different people, but to find dignity in being who they are, despite the
traumas of the past, and often cruel realities of the present.

In 2024, I attended a dance performance on the *Intrepid*, a
decommissioned aircraft carrier that is now a floating air and
space museum in New York City. The performance, written and
choreographed by marine vet Román Baca, comprised a series
of pieces about typical soldier experiences—leaving loved ones
behind, witnessing terrible combat scenes, writing letters home.
Baca had been a dancer before joining up after 9/11. He knew what
he was doing, and so did the dancers, who expertly conveyed
the harmonious grace and traumatic upheavals of military life.
But three-quarters of the way through the show, about a dozen
real veterans, wearing identical black T-shirts, arrived onstage.
There were fat ones and thin ones, tall ones and short ones,
Black, Brown, and white ones. They weren't great dancers, but
there was something poignant about these motley Americans—
arms waving, legs flying—being themselves, together onstage.

"They are all rhythm; we are all melody," a white visitor to
Africa once told me. It was a shallow generalization, but within
it was a truer one. The art of communitarian, pre-capitalist
societies—European, Asian, African, or whatever—tends to
be about the group: origin myths, totems, symbolic carvings

114 of gods. Their music is for everyone to dance and sing to, and everything they do is a work of art: the ingenious sleds and harpoons of the Inuit, the outrigger canoes of the Micronesians, the icons and churches of the Russian countryside, and even the fine craftsmanship of some twentieth-century American manufactured goods.

Today, art—that of the West, and increasingly the rest of the world—tends to emphasize the individual human voice, striving, and sometimes, almost, but never quite, succeeding, to speak to everyone else, in order to find connection with those long-ago rhythms from our collective past.

Conclusion

The hypothesis of this book is that suicide epidemics appear wherever a culture based on mutual aid, respect, and belonging suddenly gives way to a world of anonymous market transactions, individualism, and formal institutions, and, at the same time, a demonstrative love culture is weak. In such circumstances, people are forced to deal with the conundrum of the self and identity alone, without cultural guide rails or the ballast of strong affective ties. While I cannot prove that every incidence of bureaucratic marketization has resulted in a suicide crisis, the latter does seem to follow the former in every case I've been able to identify, and global surveys generally confirm that suicide is less common in societies characterized as collective compared to those characterized as individualistic. Societies in transition from the latter to the former may be the most suicidogenic of all. In addition to the examples discussed in the preceding chapters, suicide epidemics have also occurred among farmers in the US, South America, and India—not among very poor subsistence cultivators who live more or less

116   in the old ways, but among cash crop growers whose livelihoods
       are constantly threatened by arbitrary price manipulations and
       crushing bank loans that families must shoulder alone. Suicide
       also soared among Australian aborigines, Norwegian Sami,
       Irish Travellers, and other indigenous groups after they, like
       the Inuit and Micronesians, were forced virtually overnight to
       adapt to consumerist ways of life based on the nuclear family,
       the job, and the town.

       The causes of rising suicides among Black American youths
       are still under investigation, but a similar spike occurred in the
       1970s. It was concentrated among the more highly educated and
       those who had moved to other states. Sociologist Robert Davis
       speculated that, as middle-class Black families become more
       nuclearized and detached from kin and community, young peo-
       ple dealing with racism as well as their own ups and downs were
       less likely to find support in those around them and became
       more likely to blame themselves for their misfortunes.

       Contemporary high suicide groups all seem to be losing
       what the nineteenth-century German sociologist Ferdinand
       Tönnies called Gemeinschaft, which roughly translates as
       "community." Tönnies was born in 1855 into a family of wealthy
       farmers. When he was ten, they all moved to the town, where
       Tönnies's father became a merchant banker. Like his contem-
       porary, the French scholar of suicide Emile Durkheim, Tönnies's
       subject was the effect of rapid modernization on Europe's peo-
       ple. In his 1887 book *Gemeinschaft und Gesellschaft* (*Community
       and Society*), he describes how, as the village gave way to the city,
       the world of kin was replaced by a world of strangers; norms of
       generosity and mutual obligation were replaced by norms of
       greed and competition; relations between rich and poor shifted

from solicitous paternalism to frank exploitation; and craftmanship inspired by shared memories and local meanings was replaced by the mass production of utilitarian objects and art for sale to the highest bidder, regardless of whether the bidder knew anything about the artist's intentions or not.

The Gemeinschaft of the village, at least in its ideal form, if not always in reality, was based on cooperation among relatives and friends and the benign patronage relationships of landowners and peasants. Stability was maintained through moral conventions never written down that valorize decency and generosity and condemn stinginess and cruel and corrupt behavior. The Gesellschaft of cities was based on the sale of commodities and labor, and stability was maintained by contracts, police, courts, prisons, and armies.

Traditional Gemeinschaft communities have their problems, including, all too often, strict gender norms and racial and ethnic prejudices. Much of Western narrative art, from Shakespeare's *Romeo and Juliet* to Elia Kazan's *On the Waterfront* to Ralph Ellison's *Invisible Man* to Shirley Jackson's *The Lottery,* is about people trying to escape being smothered or worse by the Gemeinschaft cultures they were born into. But for many people, Gemeinschaft cultures have at least one major advantage: If we play our roles properly, they protect us from contemplation, the terror of loneliness, and the penalty of having to think about whether life is worth the struggle. In a Gemeinschaft community, we don't really belong to ourselves alone, so these questions are less likely to arise.

Gesellschaft societies, which prevail just about everywhere these days—are freer and more inclusive, but they are also colder and lonelier. Where Gemeinschaft people find their identities

118   largely through others, Gesellschaft people must search for it
        within themselves, and contemplate the haunting possibil-
        ity that their inner lives, their feelings, may not really matter to
        anyone else.

        Tönnies's worry was that the shift from Gemeinschaft/
        community/village to Gesellschaft/society/city would lead to
        rebellion and revolution. He and Durkheim knew of each other's
        work, and disagreed on points of interpretation too arcane to
        describe here. But they were witnessing and writing about the
        same thing: the disintegration of community, which is also the
        subject of this book.

        Economic growth has brought us many enjoyable and labor-
        saving goods. But as the examples discussed in this book—
        and others—show, mental health suffers when societies come to
        place greater emphasis on material goods than on relationships.
        I'm not the first to notice this. Philosophers have contemplated
        the psychological effects of monetization for almost as long as
        philosophers have existed. In his encyclopedic study *Debt: The
        First 5,000 Years*, anthropologist David Graeber traces a series of
        market transitions in societies around the world, boiling them
        down to a change in the meaning of wealth brought about by
        the introduction of coinage, commercialism, and eventually
        capitalism. Graeber doesn't use the words *Gemeinschaft* and
        Gesellschaft, but in what he calls "human economies"—roughly
        corresponding to Tönnies's Gemeinschaft communities—
        individuals are valued according to their relationships with
        each other; in commercial economies—roughly corresponding
        to Tönnies's Gesellschaft societies—people are valued accord-
        ing to their material possessions. For most of human history,
        we all lived in a human/Gemeinschaft world, in which we were

surrounded by people we could rely on to help us, and whom
we helped in return whenever we could. In these communities,
debt—what we owed others—was essentially symbolic and
infinite; no one calculated who owed what to whom. Good people gave things away; trust, decency, and generosity were the
ultimate commodities, without which everyone was doomed.

It's perhaps a sentimental picture, but as I was reading
Graeber's *Debt*, I was brought back to my years as a development
worker in Uganda some decades ago, when most Ugandans still
lived off the land in small villages. It wasn't the Garden of Eden;
there was poverty, disease, and petty corruption, but I always
knew that people would try to help me in a pinch, and even as a
stranger, I never felt alone. Much has changed in Uganda since
then. As more and more people have been drawn into the city
and the market, people became meaner, corruption—especially
among government elites—flourished, and my friends say they
feel far less safe. The suicide rate has also risen sharply.

In *Debt*, Graeber writes, the introduction of coinage and
commercialism throughout history has transformed debt
from something that holds us together to something that
both sets us free and drives us apart. Societies in which everyone was once expected to consider the well-being of others have evolved into those in which everyone is preoccupied
with the well-being of themselves and their immediate family, and debt—once the bedrock of community—has become
private and shameful. In this new, impersonal, starkly quantified transactional world, you could be imprisoned, enslaved,
or killed if you didn't pay your debts. Your daughters could be
forced into prostitution, and your sons press-ganged into the
military. It no longer mattered where anything came from or

120 who the parties to a transaction were, or whether their relationship had a future. Now debts, rather than conferring a sense of belonging, created panic; people have been known to commit horrible crimes—including murder—just to get out from under them. Modern forms of debt turn us, Graeber writes, into the very savages we falsely imagine supposedly primitive people to be.

Even those Gesellschaft/commercial people who aren't driven mad by debt are forced to grapple with the sense of self, which they must find not in foreordained community roles, but through the lottery of birth, serendipity, effort, connivance, and the sometimes-fragile ties of family and friendship. It can leave even the strongest of us plagued by doubts.

The Gemeinschaft/Gesellschaft transition occurred in spurts, at different times and places around the world. The first major shift probably began in what German philosopher Karl Jaspers called the Axial Age, roughly 800 to 200 BCE. In a famous 1948 essay in the magazine *Commentary*, Jaspers notes that, during this period, a disparate group of prophets emerged all around the world who began questioning, seemingly for the first time, the meaning of existence. These thinkers, who included Confucius and Laozi in China; the Buddha and the Jainist Vardhamana Mahavira in India; Pythagoras and Plato in Greece; Zoroaster in Iran; the prophets Elijah, Jeremiah, and Isaiah in Palestine—were the first to become "aware of consciousness itself," writes Jaspers. "The fact of thought became itself an object of thought," bringing people "face to face with the abyss ... [and] the absolute in the depth of selfhood."

Jaspers doesn't explain why these parallel spiritual awakenings occurred at around the same time in societies that were ignorant of each other, but Graeber observes that the Axial Age philosophers all lived in imperial states and were writing around the time of the introduction of coinage, which had been necessary to raise money for military campaigns. Imperial soldiers, after all, need to be paid not in goats and pumpkins and implicit Gemeinschaft mutual obligations, but in currencies that can be easily carried and stored and recognized throughout the realm.

The new coins had moral implications, in that they created entirely new categories of human relationships based on cold, quantified transactions, not gifts, favors, and symbols of fellowship. The Axial Age philosophers, Graeber writes, all placed value on things that were the "antithesis of market logic": compassion for the Buddhists, decency and filial piety for the Confucians, mysticism and the permanence of the soul for the Pythagoreans, and so on. They also shared an emphasis on charity, as if they were trying to claw back community mores that were rapidly being lost as new economic systems threatened to transform nearly all human relationships into heartless exchanges. "What value do we have to one another?" these philosophers seemed to be asking. "Or even to ourselves?"

Charles Taylor's magisterial *Sources of the Self* also traces this inward transition through the works of philosophers from Plato onward. But perhaps because he was writing during the early 1990s, a triumphalist time for capitalism, he shied away from attributing it to socioeconomic forces and the spread of markets, money, industry, and empire, even suggesting that

122   spontaneously developing self-consciousness might in some cases have furthered economic change. Whatever the case, the change was probably the most radical, and if the thesis of this book has some truth in it, the most devastating in the mental history of humanity. It's hard to imagine that it would have occurred without compulsion by the strong against the weak.

The best-studied Gemeinschaft/Gesellschaft transition occurred in Europe, during the Industrial Revolution. In 1786, David Ricardo, one of the founders of the scholarly field of liberal economics, joined his father on the London Stock Exchange as an apprentice. He was fourteen years old. Seven years later, he went into business for himself. By age thirty, he'd amassed an enormous fortune, and like many rich people, he felt he'd been gifted with unique insights, not only into moneymaking, but also into the proper administration of society. During his short lifetime, the British economy had been beset with wild swings of inflation, crop failures, gluts, and other upheavals. He was four when Adam Smith published *The Wealth of Nations*, and the two never met, but the book—which described for the first time the wealth-generating power of the free market, unconstrained by government control—made an impression on Ricardo. He went on to elaborate on Smith's ideas in a series of pamphlets and magazine essays on free trade, the labor market, and land rents.

Ricardo died at just fifty-one from an infection, but in the last twenty years of his life, he helped midwife a lasting idea: that the market, like the natural world, is subject to immutable laws analogous to the laws of physics or the (yet to be discovered) laws of biological evolution. With a bit of trimming and adjusting, the market itself would assure economic stability

through the millions of everyday supply-and-demand transactions that summed up the worth of everything, and everyone, down to the penny. The key to it all was self-interest: the
deracinated, abstract individual seeking to make himself as
rich as possible. The laissez-faire policies advocated by Smith,
Ricardo, and other early economists were astonishingly effective, in some ways. Beginning in the early nineteenth century
the European economy grew rapidly. The grand shopping bou-
levard, the department store, and the fashion show all owe their
origins to this period.

Karl Marx was among the first to articulate the problems.
It wasn't just that self-regulating market capitalism pushed
many, if not most, workers into meaningless, alienating jobs
at subsistence wages. It wasn't just that poverty and inequality were driving huge numbers of people into destitution. It was
also wrecking everything we hold dear. In a human economy,
"you can exchange love only for love, trust only for trust," he
wrote in 1844. In a market economy, even these things were for
sale. "He who can buy bravery is brave, though he be a coward."
This is what Marx meant by the famous line in *The Communist
Manifesto*, "All that is solid melts into air."

In the midst of World War II, the brilliant anthropologist Karl Polanyi picked up where Marx left off. A Jew forced
to flee his native Hungary, Polanyi struggled to understand
the growth of fascism. Why had so much of the world—not
just Germany, Italy, and Japan, but large sections of the Allied
nations too—reverted to vicious tribalism? It was, Polanyi
maintained, a desperate, misguided reaction to the existential
terror unleashed by the self-regulating, self-interest-based
market, which had caused not only a global depression and

124 widespread immiseration, but was also destroying the soul of the world.

"It was not that [the worker] was paid too little," Polanyi writes, "or even that he labored too long—though both happened often to excess—but that he was now existing under the physical conditions that denied the human shape of life." Communities in which people had once fed, clothed, and sheltered one another out of a concern for mutual survival and a sense of shared humanity were now just groups of workers in a labor market; land, once a virtually infinite resource for hunting, gathering, grazing, and planting, was fenced off, rented, bought, and sold; money, once a convenience for buying and selling, was now itself subject to a growing variety of markets that could generate interest on their own.

The result was social dislocation and alienation: the worker's reduced standing in his community, the loss of his dignity and self-respect, the deterioration of his arts and folk traditions, the fragmentation of his family, the degradation of his natural environment and his relationship to it.

The self-regulating market might make some people rich, but it also turned workers and capitalists alike into "crude, callous beings," Polanyi wrote, for whom a vicious politics of facile forms of solidarity like fascism seemed attractive.

Polanyi's anthropologist colleagues, including Margaret Mead and W. H. R. Rivers, had likewise found that indigenous groups ensnared in Western capitalist empires—from the Arctic to the American Southwest to the Pacific islands—were dying out, even where there had been no violence involved in their conquest. Wherever the self-regulating market went, it seemed to leave a trail of desolation.

Today, suicide rates globally are falling slowly, even as many
of the factors I'm pointing to—especially economic precarity—
are worsening. At the same time, more and more people, from the
post-industrial West to the sands of the Middle East, have been
turning to violent nationalism and the often-discriminatory
defense of ethnicity and religious values, as if trying to recap-
ture some bygone Gemeinschaft. Commerce, it was hoped,
would be "civilizing," in that it raises the cost of warfare. But by
decentering people from their roots, it may also be stirring up
the emotional storms that are contributing to the growing violence of our world today.

Money, markets, and capitalism forced upon human beings a
new identity, that of the individual, and we've been burdened
with the psychological fallout ever since. The world religions,
including Christianity, Judaism, Hinduism, Buddhism, and
Islam, provide a scaffolding, but they can't ultimately deliver us
from this howlingly lonely and unpredictable world, or help us
find a sure way of navigating the myriad emotional storms we
encounter in our increasingly complicated lives.

Now that we are here, what can we do about this? Perhaps our
greatest error has been to search for solutions precisely where
the problem is: within the individual. It may be no coincidence
that the Industrial Revolution—which brought commercialism into the countryside across the Western world, launching a
century-long suicide spike—was also rich in philosophers who
pondered the meaning of subjectivity and the perils of having
to negotiate a world of endless scary choices with insufficient
moral and emotional signposts. Arthur Schopenhauer, inspired
by Eastern religions, urged his readers to manage the forces

126   of the will by cultivating an attitude of detachment. Søren
Kierkegaard pondered the question of how to deal with anxiety, desire, and other overwhelming feelings, and found some
solace in inward reflection. Friedrich Nietzsche asked readers
to question everything—their morality, and what they thought
they knew—urging them to see the world with their own eyes,
as it really was. All of these thinkers eschewed the metaphysical
in favor of the contemplation of self as the soul's only real com-
pass. It was the internal voice that mattered. There was no thing
out there—no God or other abstract archetype cared about us.
Despair came to be seen as the essential characteristic of modern human beings.

Since the Industrial Revolution threw, first Americans and
Europeans, and now everyone else, back upon themselves, people began gobbling up novels—a new art form—as if desperate
to understand how fictional characters coped with the vicissi-
tudes of love, sex, and class (Jane Austen, Samuel Richardson,
Thomas Hardy, Honoré de Balzac, and countless others); being
dehumanized by poverty (Charles Dickens, Victor Hugo, etc.);
the absurdity of modern life (Franz Kafka, Jean-Paul Sartre,
Albert Camus); and so on.

On the heels of the novelists arrived the first modern
psychologists—William James, Sigmund Freud, and their many
followers—who endeavored to develop a science to explain our
anxieties and a language to explore this new kind of personal
existential suffering.

But when it comes to suicide, the inward gaze will only get
us so far. All of the suicide-prone societies I've come across
have strong traditions of stoicism. Faced with finding food
and shelter in their harsh wintry environment, the Inuit had

little use for the self-reflection that Nietzsche, Schopenhauer, Kierkegaard, Freud, and others placed their faith in. They have also been slow to see the benefits of modern psychotherapy, as have the Micronesians and other indigenous groups. Even pre-transition Russians, despite their rich literary history, had the notion of the self largely drummed out of them by Soviet masters who ordered them to strive for the glorious communist future, not to live for themselves. The gritty, masculine norms of the American working class and military are also well-known. But without a language for talking about the self and feelings, such people risk being emotionally overwhelmed by the dramas of modern life—from the often hidden abuses of the nuclear family to school bullying to mean bosses to the calamities of sudden illness, impoverishment, and bereavement. Gemeinschaft/human communities had ritual solutions to these problems, but those old scripts have less relevance and meaning for the diverse and novel problems of modern life. All too often, we are forced to face them alone. The philosophers and psychologists theorized that we could reason our way out of our emotional troubles, but that hasn't worked out as well as hoped, in part because trauma tends to shut down the very parts of the brain that help us organize and express our thoughts, even as it floods us with unbearable and confusing emotions.

Today, a new generation of doctors, psychologists, and journalists is attempting to link modern culture to our deteriorating mental health. Journalist Johann Hari's *Lost Connections* describes how modernity has robbed us of the things worth living for, including friendship, solidarity, meaningful work, and mutual respect and understanding. In *The Anxious Generation*, social psychologist Jonathan Haidt laments the loss of the

128   playfulness of childhood to social media, computer games, and
overprotective parenting. In *The Myth of Normal*, doctor Gabor
Maté and his writer son, Daniel, identify such modern forms of
trauma as overmedicalized childbirth practices, punitive childrearing conventions, bullying by peers, consumerism, and other
modern compulsions that neglect the emotional needs of parents and children and alienate us from each other.

This latest group of authors recognizes that we need to
look not only within ourselves, but also to our policymakers for
answers. We all have a need to feel useful to others, and that need
will only be fulfilled when we find a way to build a world with
a place for everyone. Unfortunately, when policymakers and
their advisors have taken a stab at it, they've tended to miss this
point. In his 2018 book *Why Liberalism Failed*, Patrick Deneen,
like Vice President J. D. Vance and many other political conservatives, blames our current state of social disintegration on the
freedoms unleashed by liberation movements and selfish individualism. What we need, these thinkers say, are government
policies that encourage a return to homespun values, including
religious observance, and duty to family and community. There
is nothing wrong with those values, but it's virtually impossible
to create a sense of community from the outside, by urging people to stay married to partners they feel estranged from, or to go
to church when they aren't observant, or to participate in group
activities they don't care about, or to make friends when they
feel that no one could possibly understand them.

I suggest Deneen, Vance, and the others spend a week, or
even a day, working on the floor of a Walmart or at an Amazon
warehouse. Then let them tell us what they think the root of
the problems is. Is it really that our political system has led

ordinary people into a mire of self-indulgence? Or, as Deneen's critic Robert Kuttner suggests, is the lack of self-discipline and sense of community mostly all on the side of the corporate class, whose power has been allowed to hypertrophy precisely because of the erosion of the checks and balances that were supposed to be built into political liberalism in the first place? Even many liberals don't get this. As harsh US labor policies were tearing America's communities apart in the 1990s and 2000s, both the Clinton and Obama White Houses held conferences on declining social capital. Unfortunately, their recommendations tended to stress changing the behaviors of individuals, urging them, for example, to join groups or make friends. It hasn't worked.

Communities do form spontaneously, if the conditions are right. The best policy I can think of is to strive for greater economic equality, which will naturally reduce insecurity, and, in turn, foster greater spiritual as well as material generosity. When positive communities begin to emerge, the trick then is not to ruin them. The communities that give me hope formed across ethnic lines. In *Secondhand Time*, her literary history of the collapse of the Soviet Union, Svetlana Alexievich interviews Margarita, a middle-aged Armenian who grew up in Soviet-era Azerbaijan. She tells Svetlana Alexievich, "[E]veryone lived together like one big family, Azerbaijanis, Russians, Armenians, Ukrainians, Tatars." On special holidays, there was a huge feast with food and wine from everywhere: Russian blinis, Georgian khinkali, tea with cinnamon and cardamom. "Anyone could go into anyone else's house—and everyone would be welcomed as a guest." The most glamorous woman she knew was an Armenian air hostess who was married to an Azerbaijani taxi

130   driver. "I don't remember any discussion of their nationalities. The world was divided up differently: is someone a good or bad person, are they greedy or kind?"

After the USSR was dissolved, Azerbaijan declared independence and then its Armenian community declared independence from Azerbaijan. A brutal war broke out, in part over control of the region's vast oil and mineral wealth. That war simmers to this day. Alexievich's wistful informant had to hide out from Azerbaijani gangs, one of which mugged and beat her Azerbaijani husband because he had an Armenian wife. It was the specter of profit that wrecked everything. Money, writes the philosopher Simone Weil, "destroys human roots wherever it is able to penetrate, [because it] manages to outweigh other motives."

Communities have emerged in America, too, without the Leviathan of Soviet communism, but they have often done so amid the struggle against those aspects of capitalism that are most harmful. One glimmer of hope—in the US, at least—is the fledgling regrowth of the US labor movement. If it succeeds, it could improve not only the financial health of US workers, but their mental health as well.

America's unions were once a binding force in working-class communities. When General Electric workers struck for higher wages in the 1940s, cooks at nearby restaurants prepared free meals for them and college students joined them on the picket lines, along with veterans, American Legionnaires, and even policemen. The odd senator and congressman also cheered them on.[*]

* Kim Phillips-Fein, *Invisible Hands: The Making of the Conservative Movement from the New Deal to Reagan* (Norton, 2009).

GE eventually conceded to the workers' demands but then set out to avoid a repeat by hiring lobbyists and consultants to chip away at rights guaranteed under the 1935 National Labor Relations Act. "Right to work" contract clauses now meant companies could hire nonunion workers, interrogate employees about union activities, search their bags to see if they were carrying union literature (a fireable offense in many cases) and force everyone to attend meetings at which free enterprise was praised and unions criticized, with no opportunity for pro-union speakers to respond.[*] Threats, bribes, and other violations of union activists' rights increased, but were rarely prosecuted.

Ronald Reagan, once a staunch Democrat whose family had benefited from Depression-era New Deal programs, went to work as a spokesman for GE in 1954. When he became president in 1981, he took the opportunity to fire some eleven thousand striking air traffic controllers. The corporate class found this so admirable, it's now taught as a case study in US business schools.[†] Unionized meatpackers, bus drivers, paper mill workers, copper miners, and others were soon subject to a new strikebreaking craze, and the number of strikes—virtually the only real leverage workers have—fell steeply, along with union membership, which now stands at 10 percent of the American workforce, compared to 90 percent in France.[‡]

[*] Barbara Ehrenreich, "Lexus and the Right to Pee," in *The Age of Inequality: Corporate America's War on Working People*, edited by Jeremy Gantz (Verso, 2017).

[†] Andrew Storm, "Ronald Reagan Has Shaped U.S. Labor Law for Decades," *OnLabor*, January 4, 2024.

[‡] Steven Greenhouse, *Beaten Down, Worked Up: The Past, Present, and Future of American Labor* (Knopf, 2017).

132   At the turn of the twentieth century, countless workers lost
their lives to factory and mining accidents and Pinkerton bul-
lets. But they seldom died by their own hand. What they had
that today's workers lack is solidarity, born out of shared struggle. By contrast, today's workers have been demoralized not
only by a corporate culture that is well prepared to thwart them,
but also by a prevailing discourse of condescension, in which
their problems are blamed, not on the companies that exploit
them, but on supposedly nefarious labor leaders, and their own
personal failure to embrace the American Dream.*

Lynn Nottage's fictional 2015 play *Sweat*, which is based on real
events, opens with two women, one Black, one white, dancing
in a Pennsylvania Rust Belt bar. They are factory workers and
best friends. One day, they are told that a management job has
just opened up and the factory is planning to hire from the shop
floor. They both apply and the Black woman gets it, but soon
realizes she's been hired to downsize, and eventually close, the
factory, which is moving to Mexico where labor is cheaper. The
whole community is destroyed. The two women end up hating
each other; one becomes an addict, the other an impoverished
home health aide. Both of their sons end up in jail, and the bar-
tender ends up with a broken skull. That's how you destroy a
community. That's how you create racial enmity.

     But all is not lost. Communities can regrow, just like dec-
imated forests. Making families and people in general more
financially secure would definitely help. We are kinder to

*Michael Sandel, *The Tyranny of Merit: What's Become of the Common Good?*
(Farrar, Straus and Giroux, 2020); J.D. Vance, *Hillbilly Elegy: A Memoir of a
Family and Culture in Crisis* (Harper, 2016).

one another when we don't feel threatened. Otherwise, the best advice I can think of is not to make things worse, not to destroy Gemeinschaft where it exists. Let's treat communities like ecosystems so that every time a major economic policy shift is proposed—a massive new trade deal or development project—the effects on communities are considered, and the preservation of Gemeinschaft is prioritized. Ideally, studies of this, analogous to the environmental impact studies now required by all World Bank loans to developing countries, would be conducted with the full and meaningful involvement of affected communities.

British prime minister Margaret Thatcher famously maintained that there was no "society"—by which she meant essential community, that collective property of human beings Tönnies called Gemeinschaft. No, Thatcher insisted, there were only individuals and families, and government policy should focus on making as many of them as possible as rich as possible. For the business class of the go-go 1980s, it seemed refreshingly obvious; for Britain's struggling labor unions and soon-to-be demolished factory towns, it seemed grotesque and heartless.

In 1888, Emile Durkheim, the father of suicide studies, wrote that, according to classical economists like Smith and Ricardo, "there is nothing real in society except the individual; it is from him that everything emanates and it is to him that everything returns." It was, he concluded, "a sad portrait of the pure egoist." Not only were real people subject to countless influences of time, place, family, religion, and other variables, there was also, Durkheim maintained, a social quantity, a thing that affects us all but is a characteristic of the group and not of

134   any one person alone. Without it, he went on to demonstrate in
his classic study of suicide, we are lost.

If writing this book has convinced me of anything, it is that
Thatcher and her economist kin, though right about much, were
wrong about community/Gemeinschaft or whatever you want
to call it, and Durkheim was right. We are losing something, and
even though we can't see or measure it, many of us, especially
those with suicidal thoughts, feel this loss profoundly. Some
elements of it survive, even in these harsh times—in well-
functioning neighborhoods, in friendship networks, sometimes
in the military, and in some schools and workplaces. You know
it when you see it; it's where you feel your dignity is recognized.
Let's not lose what's left of it.

FURTHER READING

The following books have been of great help to me in writing this one:

ON HOLLYWOOD

Jean Stein, *West of Eden* (Random House, 2016).

ON SUICIDE

Emile Durkheim, *Suicide: A Study in Sociology* (Routledge & Kegan Paul, 1952/1897).

Maurice Halbwachs, *The Causes of Suicide* (Routledge & Kegan Paul, Henley-on-Thames, 1978).

Thomas Joiner, *Why People Die by Suicide* (Harvard University Press, 2007).

Thomas Joiner, *The Varieties of Suicidal Experience: A New Theory of Suicidal Violence* (NYU Press, 2024).

Edwin Shneidman, *The Suicidal Mind* (Oxford University Press, 1998).

Kay Redfield Jamison, *Night Falls Fast: Understanding Suicide* (Vintage, 2000).

Yossi Levi-Belz and Dafni Assaf, *Under a Dark Black Sky: Dialogues on Mental Pain, Suicide and Hope* (Hakibutz Hameuhad, 2022, in Hebrew).

ON THE INUIT

Jean Briggs, *Never in Anger: Portrait of an Eskimo Family* (Harvard University Press, 1970).

Michael Kral, *The Return of the Sun: Suicide and Reclamation Among Inuit of Arctic Canada* (Oxford University Press, 2019).

Willem Rasing, *Too Many People: Contact, Disorder, Change in an Inuit Society, 1822–2015* (Nunavut Arctic College Media, 2017).

ON MICRONESIA

Catherine Lutz, *Unnatural Emotions: Everyday Sentiments on a Micronesian Atoll and Their Challenge to Western Theory* (University of Chicago Press, 1988).

136   Francis X. Hezel, *Making Sense of Micronesia: The Logic of Pacific Island Culture* (University of Hawaii Press, 2013).

David Nevin, *The American Touch in Micronesia* (Norton, 1997).

Barbara Gail Horning Demory, *An Illusion of Surplus: The Effect of Status Rivalry Upon Family Food Consumption* (PhD Thesis, University of California, Berkeley, 1976).

ON RUSSIA

Svetlana Alexievich, *Secondhand Time: The Last of the Soviets* (Random House, 2013).

Dale Pesmen, *Russia and Soul: An Exploration* (Cornell University Press, 2000).

Michelle Parsons, *Dying Unneeded: The Cultural Context of the Russian Mortality Crisis* (Vanderbilt University Press, 2014).

Masha Gessen, *The Future Is History: How Totalitarianism Reclaimed Russia* (Riverhead, 2017).

David Remnick, *Resurrection: The Struggle for a New Russia* (Penguin Random House, 1997).

Tomothy Colton, *Yeltsin: A Life* (Basic Books, 2011).

Alena Ledeneva, *Russia's Economy of Favours: Blat, Networking and Informal Exchange* (Cambridge University Press, 1998).

Nancy Reis, *Russian Talk: Culture and Conversation During Perestroika* (Cornell University Press, 1997).

Stephen Handelman, *Comrade Criminal: Russia`s New Mafiya* (Yale University Press, 1995).

David Stuckler and Sanjay Basu, *The Body Economic: Why Austerity Kills* (Basic Books, 2013).

Boris Yeltsin's three autobiographies:

Against the Grain: An Autobiography (Simon and Schuster, 1990).

The Struggle for Russia (Crown, 1994).

Midnight Diaries (Public Affairs, 2000).

ON AMERICA'S MENTAL HEALTH CRISIS   137

Barbara Ehrenreich, *Nickel and Dimed: On (Not) Getting By in America* (Picador, 2001).

Gabor and Daniel Mate, *The Myth of Normal: Trauma, Illness, and Healing in a Toxic Culture* (Avery, 2022).

Bessel Van Der Kolk, *The Body Keeps the Score: Brain, Mind, and Body in the Healing of Trauma* (Penguin, 2015).

Stephen Marglin, *The Dismal Science: How Thinking Like an Economist Undermines Community* (Harvard University Press, 2008).

Vivek Murthy, *Together: The Healing Power of Human Connection in a Sometimes Lonely World* (Harper, 2020).

Johan Hari, *Lost Connections: Uncovering the Real Causes of Depression and the Unexpected Solutions* (Bloomsbury, 2018).

Jonathan Haidt, *The Anxious Generation: How the Great Rewiring of Childhood Is Causing an Epidemic of Mental Illness* (Penguin, 2024).

Anne Case and Angus Deaton, *Deaths of Despair and the Future of Capitalism* (Princeton University Press, 2020).

Emily Guendelsberger, *On the Clock: What Low-Wage Work Did to Me and How It Drives America Insane* (Little Brown, 2019).

ON THE MENTAL HEALTH OF US VETERANS

Edward Tick, *War and the Soul: Healing Our Nation's Veterans from Post-Traumatic Stress Disorder* (Quest Books, 2005).

Edward Tick, *Warrior's Return: Restoring the Soul After War* (Sounds True, 2014).

Sebastian Junger, *Tribe: On Home-coming and Belonging* (Twelve, 2016).

ON CULTURE, ART AND SUICIDE

Clifford Geertz, *The Interpretation of Cultures* (Basic Books, 1973).

Leo Tolstoy, *What Is Art?* Translated by Aylmer Maude (Funk and Wagnalls, 1904).

Søren Kierkegaard, *Either/Or: A Fragment of Life* (Penguin, 1992).

138   Arthur Schopenhauer, *The World as Will and Representation, Vol. 1* (Echo Point Books, 2021).

Jean-Paul Sartre, *Nausea*, trans. by Robert Baldick (Penguin, 2000).

Albert Camus, *The Myth of Sisyphus*, trans. by Justin O'Brien (Vintage, 1991).

Mark Seinfelt, *Final Drafts: Suicides of World-Famous Authors* (Prometheus, 1999).

Kay Redfield Jamison, *Touched with Fire: Manic-Depressive Illness and the Artistic Temperament* (Free Press, 1996).

ON THE COSTS OF ECONOMIC TRANSFORMATION

David Graeber, *Debt: The First 5,000 Years* (Melville House, 2021).

Karl Polanyi, *The Great Transformation* (Penguin, 2024/1944).

Nicholas Lemann, *Transaction Man: The Rise of the Deal and the Decline of the American Dream* (Farrar, Strauss and Giroux, 2019).

David Weil, *The Fissured Workplace: Why Work Became So Bad for So Many and What Can Be Done to Improve It* (Harvard University Press, 2017).

David Harvey, *The Condition of Postmodernity: An Enquiry into the Origins of Cultural Change* (Wiley-Blackwell, 1991).

Kim Phillips-Fein, *Invisible Hands: The Making of the Conservative Movement from the New Deal to Reagan* (Norton, 2009).

Steven Greenhouse, *Beaten Down, Worked Up: The Past, Present, and Future of American Labor* (Knopf, 2017).

Michael Sandel, *The Tyranny of Merit: What's Become of the Common Good?* (Farrar, Straus and Giroux, 2020).

ACKNOWLEDGMENTS

I wish to thank everyone I interviewed for this book, including those who remain anonymous. Discussions with Ed Tick, David Celani, Christopher Lukas, Stephan Wolfert, Garett Reppenhagen, Wendy D'Andrea, Alisha Ali, Edward Vessel, Michael Kral, Jack Hicks, Yossi Levi-Belz, Fr. Francis Hezel, and Will Affleck were particularly helpful.

Anne Case, Angus Deaton, Jesse Ribot, and, as always, Petr Petr listened kindly as I test-drove various ideas for this book; Mary Blume, Jacob Burckhardt, Bill Easterly, Vivian Gornick, Bill Herbert, Pankaj Mishra, and Marc Ribot read over parts or all of the manuscript, catching many wrong turns. The remaining errors are, of course, on me.

I also wish to thank the Pulitzer Center on Crisis Reporting for a grant that enabled me to travel to Nunavut to research suicide among the Inuit, and Michael Shae, Emily Greenhouse, and the gang at *The New York Review of Books* for publishing the resulting article.

I thank Bard College for funds to support further research for this book and for being a great place to work and teach.

It was a pleasure to work once again with Nick Lemann, Jimmy So, Jaime Leifer, and the team at Columbia Global Reports. Thanks also to my agent, Anna Stein, for caring about this project even from its befuddled beginnings.

INTRODUCTION

8 **"Black choler":** Robert Burton, *The Anatomy of Melancholy* (1621), Project Gutenberg, https://www .gutenberg.org/ebooks/10800.

9 **"psychache," an excruciating feeling of utter loss:** Edwin Shneidman, "Suicide as Psychache: A Clinical Approach to Self-Destructive Behavior, *Journal of Nervous and Mental Disease* 181, no. 3 (1993): 145–147; Edwin Shneidman, *The Suicidal Mind*, revised ed. (Oxford University Press, 1998).

9 **no way to predict who will die by suicide:** Matthew Michael Large, "The Role of Prediction in Suicide Prevention," *Dialogues in Clinical Neuroscience* 20, no. 3 (2018): 197–205, https://doi.org/10.31887 /DCNS.2018.20.3/mlarge.

9 **only about one in a thousand of them take their own lives in any given year:** In 2023, forty-six million US adults had depression, and fifty thousand died by suicide.

9 **measures that really do save lives:** Thomas Joiner, John Kalafat, John Draper, Heather Stokes, Marshall Knudson, Alan L. Berman, and Richard McKeon, "Establishing Standards for the Assessment of Suicide Risk Among Callers to the National Suicide Prevention Lifeline," *Suicide and Life-Threatening Behavior* 37, no. 3 (2007): 353–365; J. John Mann, Alan Apter, Jose Bertolote et al., "Suicide Prevention Strategies: A Systematic Review," *JAMA* 294, no. 16 (2005): 2064–2074. S. Briggs et al., "The Effectiveness of Psychoanalytic/ Psychodynamic Psychotherapy for Reducing Suicide Attempts and Self-Harm: Systematic Review and Meta-Analysis," *British Journal of Psychiatry* 214, no. 6 (June 2019): 320-328; M. Sarchiapone, L. Mandelli, M. Iosue, C. Andrisano, A. Roy, "Controlling Access to Suicide Means," *International Journal of Environmental Research and Public Health* 8 (2011): 4550–4562.

10 **have faith anyway:** Søren Kierkegaard, *The Sickness Unto Death: A Christian Psychological Exposition for Upbuilding and Awakening* (1849) (Princeton University Press, 1983).

10 **embrace voluntary death if you want to:** Paolo Stellino, "Nietzsche on Suicide," *Nietzsche-Studien* 42, no. 1 (2013): 151–177; Friedrich Nietzsche, *Thus Spoke Zarathustra: A Book for Everyone and No One* (Penguin 1961).

10 **find pleasure in the little things in life:** Albert Camus, *The Myth of Sisyphus and Other Essays* (Vintage, 1955).

10 **just do something and don't worry about what it all means:** Jean Paul Sartre, *Nausea* (1938) (New Directions, 2013).

10 **because they think no one cares about them:** Thomas Joiner, *Why People Die by Suicide* (Harvard University Press, 2005).

10 **a force of nature that distorts people's minds so they become convinced that they are a burden to others:** "The Suicide of Democracy?" (ft. Dr. Thomas Joiner), *Out of the Box with Jonathan Russo*, Season 2, Ep. 11 (Monday, June 12, 2023); Thomas Joiner, *Why People Die by Suicide*; Edwin Schniedman, *The Suicidal Mind*.

11 **most common trigger for suicide is a perceived rupture in a close relationship:** Michael Kral, *The Return of the Sun: Suicide and Social Transformation Among Inuit in Arctic Canada* (Oxford University Press, 2019); Francis X. Hezel, "Suicide and the Micronesian Family," *Contemporary Pacific* 1, nos. 1–2 (1989): 43–74, http://hdl.handle.net/10125/8356.

11 **inordinately common among people who die by suicide:** Kay Redfield Jameison, *Night Falls Fast: Understanding Suicide* (Vintage, 2010); Kees van Heeringen, *The Neuroscience of Suicidal Behavior* (Cambridge University Press, 2018); Jesse Bering, *Suicidal: Why We Kill Ourselves* (University of Chicago Press, 2018).

11 **been shown to double or even triple suicide attempts:** Tyra Lagerberg, Anthony A. Matthews, Nanbo Zhu, et al., "Effect of Selective Serotonin Reuptake Inhibitor Treatment Following Diagnosis of Depression on Suicidal Behaviour Risk: A Target Trial Emulation," *Neuropsychopharmacology* 48, no. 12 (2023): 1760–1768, https://doi.org/10.1038/s41386-023-01676-3.

12 **suicides nearly tripled in Belgium, Italy, and France, and quadrupled in Austria:** Robert Nye, *Crime, Madness, and Politics in Modern France: The Medical Concept of National Decline* (Princeton University Press, 1984); Maurice Halbwachs, *The Causes of Suicide* (Routledge, 1978); Marzio Barbagli, *Farewell to the World: A History of Suicide*, trans. Lucinda Byatt (Polity, 2015).

12 **young veterans of the Iraq and Afghan wars:** *Suicide Among Veterans and Other Americans 2001–2014*, Veterans Administration Office of Mental Health and Suicide Prevention, 2016 (updated August 2017). See table 5 and Figure 22.

12 **doubled among middle-aged Russians after the collapse of Soviet communism:** David Stuckler and Sanjay Basu, *The Body Economic: Why Austerity Kills* (Basic Books, 2013); David A. Leon, Laurent Chenet, Vladimir M. Shkolnikov, Sergei Zakharov, Judith

142   Shapiro, Galina Rakhmanova, Sergei Vassin, and Martin McKee, "Huge Variation in Russian Mortality Rates 1984–94: Artefact, Alcohol, or What?" *The Lancet* 350, no. 9075 (1997): 383–388.

13 **after deindustrialization commenced in the 1970s:** Anne Case and Angus Deaton, *Deaths of Despair and the Future of Capitalism* (Princeton University Press, 2020), 127.

13 **suicide among Inuit youths in the Canadian Arctic soared from almost zero:** Jack Hicks, *Statistical Data on Death by Suicide by Nunavut Inuit, 1920 to 2014* (Nunavut Tunngavik Inc., 2015), https://www.tunngavik.com/files/2015/09/2015-09-14-Statistical-Historical-Suicide-Date-Eng.pdf.

13 **similar spikes commenced:** Francis X. Hezel, "Suicide and the Micronesian Family"; Mary Walker, *Suicide Among the Irish Traveller Community, 2000–2006* (Paveepoint, 2008); Dorothy Kizza, Birthe Loa Knizek, Eugene Kinyanda, and Heidi Hjelmeland, "Men in Despair: A Qualitative Psychological Autopsy Study of Suicide in Northern Uganda," *Transcultural Psychiatry* 49, no. 5 (2012): 696–717.

14 **isn't more common during wars:** David Lester, "Suicide During War and Genocides," in Danuta Wasserman, ed., *Oxford Textbook of Suicidology and Suicide Prevention,* 2nd ed. (Oxford University Press, 2021), 209–213.

14 **experienced some environmental disaster:** Kairi Kõlves, Keili E. Kõlves, and Diego De Leo, "Natural Disasters and Suicidal Behaviours: A Systematic Literature Review," *Journal of Affective Disorders* 146, no. 1 (2013): 1–14.

14 **Suicide was common among African slaves:** Terri Snyder, *The Power to Die: Slavery and Suicide in British North America* (University of Chicago Press, 2015).

14 **suicide rate of African Americans has been consistently lower than that of US whites:** See John L. Macintosh, "Trends in Racial Differences in US Suicide," *Death Studies* 13, no. 3 (1989).

14 **Jews in Nazi-occupied Europe killed themselves in large numbers:** See Marzio Barbagli, *Farewell to the World,* p. 134; and David Lester, "The Suicide Rate in the Concentration Camps Was Extraordinarily High: A Comment on Bronisch and Lester," *Archives of Suicide Research* 8, no. 2 (January 2004).

14 **their children are no more likely to die by suicide:** See Itzak Levav et al., "Psychopathology and Other Health Dimensions Among the Offspring of Holocaust Survivors: Results from the Israel National Health Survey," *The Israel*

Journal of Psychiatry and Related Sciences, February 2007.

14   **mental pain that drives suicide is really the flip side of love:** Yovell's theory is presented in the fascinating book *Under the Black Sky: Dialogues on Mental Pain, Suicide and Hope* (in Hebrew, Kibbutz Hameuhad, 2022), by the Israeli psychologist Yossi Levi-Belz and Dafni Assaf, who lost her daughter to suicide in 2007.

15   **recently experienced the loss of a close personal relationship:** Richard C. W. Hall, Dennie E. Platt, and Ryan C. W. Hall, "Suicide Risk Assessment: A Review of Risk Factors for Suicide in 100 Patients Who Made Severe Suicide Attempts: Evaluation of Suicide Risk in a Time of Managed Care," *Psychosomatics* 40 (1999): 18–27.

15   **suicide notes often express love for those left behind:** Silvia Sara Canetto and David Lester, "Love and Achievement Motives in Women's and Men's Suicide Notes," *Journal of Psychology* 136, no. 5 (2002): 573–576; Sandra Sanger and Patricia McCarthy Veach, "The Interpersonal Nature of Suicide: A Qualitative Investigation of Suicide Notes," *Archives of Suicide Research* 12, no. 4 (2008): 352–365, https://doi.org/10.1080/1381111080232 5232.

15   **were especially likely to report that in the three preceding days, they'd felt "unusually**

intense or deep feelings of love":   143
Zimri S. Yaseen, Karin Fisher, Esperanza Morales, and Igor I. Galynker, "Love and Suicide: The Structure of the Affective Intensity Rating Scale (AIRS) and Its Relation to Suicidal Behavior," *PLoS ONE* 7, no. 8 (2012): e44069, https://doi.org/10.1371/journal.pone.0044069.

15   **which they presumably also felt were not reciprocated:** Thomas Joiner, *Why People Die by Suicide*.

15   **seems to have been an outcast even among his fellow terrorists:** Adam Lankford, *The Myth of Martyrdom: What Really Drives Suicide Bombers, Rampage Shooters, and Other Self-Destructive Killers* (St. Martin's Press, 2013).

16   **the passions of youth against the onslaught of Bourgeois boredom:** Al Alvarez, *The Savage God. A Study of Suicide* (Random House, 1971), 214.

16   **searched, in vain, for a suicidogenic organ in the cadavers:** Ian Hacking, *The Taming of Chance* (Cambridge University Press, 1990).

16   **theorized that Europe's soaring suicide rate was a manifestation of a general process of moral decline:** Steven Lukes, *Emile Durkheim: His Life and Work. A Historical and Critical Study*

144 (Stanford University Press, 1985), 224, 206, 213, 207.

17 **explored through studies of hypnosis, hallucinations, and spiritualism:** Laurent Mucchielli and Marc Renneville, "Les causes du suicide: pathologie individuelle ou sociale? Durkheim, Halbwachs et les psychiatres de leur temps (1830–1930)," *Déviance et Société*, 22, no. 1 (1998): 3–36.

17 **Durkheim followed this research closely:** Laurent Mucchielli and Marc Renneville, "Les causes du suicide: pathologie individuelle ou sociale?"

17 **Nikolai Tesla:** Amanda Gefter, "Tesla's Pigeon," *Nautilus*. December 6, 2023.

17 **expressions of resolutions planted in their minds by a disintegrating society:** Laurent Mucchielliand and Marc Renneville, "Les causes du suicide: pathologie individuelle ou sociale?"

18 **a series of lectures on suicide at the University of Chicago:** Christian Topalov, "Maurice Halbwachs and Chicago Sociologists," *Revue française de sociologie* 49, supplement (2008: 187–214, https://www.cairn.info /revue-francaise-de-sociologie-1 -2008-5-page-187.htm.

18 **by the end of the semester, only three students remained:** Suzanne Vromen, "Chicago in 1930: Maurice Halbwachs' Outsider View of the City and Its Sociologists," in ed. Anthony J. Blasi, *Diverse Histories of American Sociology* (Brill Academic, 2005).

18 **he also lacked Durkheim's bias against subjectivity:** Laurent Mucchielliand and Marc Renneville, "Les causes du suicide: pathologie individuelle ou sociale?"

19 **incapable of ever finding in another any support, nor anything to replace what you have lost:** Maurice Halbwachs, 1930, quoted in Laurent Mucchielli and and Marc Renneville, "Les causes du suicide: pathologie individuelle ou sociale?"

19 **meaning of the word "lonely" changed:** See Fay Bound-Alberti, *A Biography of Loneliness* (Oxford University Press, 2019).

20 **extended family, which once formed a social mesh that supported everyone, waned in significance:** Lawrence Stone, *The Family, Sex and Marriage in England, 1500–1800* (Harper Perennial, 1977; abridged edition, 1983) and Norbert Elias, *The Civilizing Process: Sociogenetic and Psychogenetic Investigations* (Blackwell Publishing, 1939; revised edition, 2000).

21 **Only the greedy and selfish were looked down upon and excluded:** See, for example: *Atanarjuat: The Fast Runner*, a film

by Zacharias Kunuk (2003); Jean Briggs, *Never in Anger: Portrait of an Eskimo Family* (Harvard University Press, 1971); Francis X. Hezel, *Making Sense of Micronesia: The Logic of Pacific Island Culture* (University of Hawaii Press, 2013).

22 Love is not just a feeling; it's also a culture: See Lawrence Stone, *The Family, Sex and Marriage in England, 1500–1800*, for an account of how this happened at one time and place.

22 love poems, songs, and stories came to occupy the center of Western culture: Denis de Rougement, *Love in the Western World* (1939) (Princeton University Press, 1983).

22 love came to be seen as a force superior to the gods: Erich Fromm, *The Art of Loving* (1956) (Harper Perennial, 2006).

23 could sell them at markets or abandon them and marry someone else without divorcing: Lawrence Stone, *The Family, Sex and Marriage in England, 1500–1800*.

23 now promoted ideals of conjugal and parental love: Jean Flandrin, *Families in Former Times: Kinship, Household and Sexuality* (Cambridge University Press, 1979).

23 That was love, and according to accounts of anthropologists: Marcel Mauss, *The Gift: Forms and Functions of Exchange in Archaic*

Societies (1925) (Martino Fine Books, 2011).

24 she published a haunting oral history: Jean Stein, *West of Eden: An American Place* (Random House, 2017).

25 in nearly every case, they'd been haunted by "the loss of childhood's special joys": Edwin S. Shneidman, *The Suicidal Mind*.

25 "The early dawn" would see their two mothers pouring the first martinis: Jean Stein, *West of Eden: An American Place* (Random House 2016).

CHAPTER 1

27 The research for this chapter was supported by the Pulitzer Center on Crisis Reporting.

27 Sam was making toast: Because of the sensitive nature of this material, most Inuit sources asked that their real names not be used.

28 would have the highest suicide rate in the world: Danuta Wasserman, Qi Cheng, and Guo-Xin Jiang, "Global Suicide Rates Among Young People Aged 15–19," *World Psychiatry* 4, no. 2 (2005): 114–120; Jack Hicks, *Statistical Data on Death by Suicide by Nunavut Inuit, 1920 to 2014*.

28 Almost one-third of Nunavut Inuit have attempted suicide: L. J. Kirmayer, M. Malus,

146   and L. J. Boothroyd, "Suicide
Attempts Among Inuit Youth: A
Community Survey of Prevalence
and Risk Factors," *Acta Psychiatrica
Scandinavia* 94, no. 1 (1996): 8–17;
Michael J. Kral, "The Weight on
Our Shoulders Is Too Much and We
Are Falling," *Medical Anthropology
Quarterly* 27, no. 1 (2013): 63–83,
http://dx.doi.org/10.1111/maq
.12016.

28   **suicide was rare, and among
young people, almost unknown:**
During the 1960s, anthropologist
Asen Balicki reported a very high
suicide rate among the Inuit of Pelly
Bay, a community where he carried
out ethnographic research over
several years. However, according
to suicide expert Jack Hicks, there
is no evidence to support this
claim in the detailed records of the
Royal Canadian Mounted Police,
missionaries, or the coroner's
office. See Jack Hicks, *Statistical
Data on Death by Suicide by Nunavut
Inuit, 1920 to 2014.*

29   **swarms of mosquitoes can
exsanguinate a caribou:** Brooks
Hays, "Climate Change a Boon
for Arctic Mosquitoes," UPI,
September 16, 2015, https://www
.upi.com/Science_News/2015/09
/16/Climate-change-a-boon-for
-arctic-mosquitoes/6461442
420878/.

29   **"The different families
appear always to live on good
terms with each other":** Referred
to in Willem Rasing, *Too Many
People: Contact, Disorder and Change
in the High Arctic* (Nunavut Arctic
College, 2017).

30   **if that didn't work, singing
duels might be organized:**
Penelope Eckett and Russell
Newmark, "Central Eskimo Song
Duels: A Contextual Analysis of
Ritual Ambiguity," *Ethnology* 19,
no. 2 (1980): 191–211.

30   **used only as a last resort
against those whose behavior
endangered others:** Kenn Harper,
*Thou Shalt Do No Murder: Inuit,
Injustice, and the Canadian Arctic*
(Nunavut Arctic College, 2017).

30   **homicide, domestic violence,
child abuse, vandalism, and
alcoholism:** Steve Ducharme,
"Iqaluit Ranks Near the Top
for Violence Against Women,"
Nunatsiaq News, January 30, 2018,
https://nunatsiaq.com/stories
/article/65674iqaluit_ranks
_near_the_top_for_violence
_against_women/; Emma Tranter,
"Declare Child Sexual Abuse a
Crisis, Nunavut MLA Demands of
Premier," *Nunatsiaq News,* June 10,
2019, https://nunatsiaq.com
/stories/article/declare-child
-sexual-abuse-a-crisis-nunavut
-mla-demands-of-premier/;
Mike Gibbins, "Alcohol-Related
Hospitalizations in N.W.T. 5 Times
National Rate," CBC News, June 22,
2017, https://www.cbc.ca/news
/canada/north/alcohol-related

-hospitalizations-nwt-5-times
-national-1.4172897; "Northern
Territories Had Highest Crime
Rates, Severity in Canada in 2017,"
CBC News, September 9, 2018,
https://www.cbc.ca/news/canada
/north/northern-territories
-highest-crime-rate-severity
-1.4815397; Nunavut and Canada
Homicides, 1999–2017.

30   **over half the population uses
drugs:** Willem Rasing, *Too Many
People*.

31   **who collected testimonies for
an Inuit-initiated inquiry into the
dog killings:** "Analysis of the RCMP
Sled Dog Report," Qikiqtani Truth
Commission Thematic Reports and
Special Studies, 1950–1975 (2014),
https://www.qtcommission.ca
/sites/default/files/public
/thematic_reports/thematic
_reports_english_rcmp_sled_dog
.pdf.

32   **surrendered them in tears:**
Daniel Schwartz, "Truth and
Reconciliation Commission: By the
Numbers," CBC News, June 2, 2015,
https://www.cbc.ca/news
/indigenous/truth-and
-reconciliation-commission-by
-the-numbers-1.3096185.

32   **Canadian officials admitted
that the schools' effect on
aboriginal cultures amounted to
a form of genocide:** Jane Cohen,
"Residential School System Was
'Cultural Genocide,' Says Report,"
Canadian Lawyer, June 2, 2015,

https://www.canadianlawyermag
.com/news/general/residential
-school-system-was-cultural
-genocide-says-report/273227.

33   **the suicide rate among young
Canadians in general remained
below 20:** Jack Hicks, *Statistical
Data on Death by Suicide by Nunavut
Inuit, 1920 to 2014*.

33   **have taken their own lives
at lower rates than US whites:**
See Marzio Barbagli, *Farewell
to the World*, p. 134; and David
Lester, "The Suicide Rate in
the Concentration Camps Was
Extraordinarily High."

33   **children of Jews in Nazi-
occupied Europe were no more
likely to die by suicide:** See Itzak
Levav et al, "Psychopathology
and Other Health Dimensions
Among the Offspring of Holocaust
Survivors."

34   **such disorders often have
social causes:** See Richard Bentall,
*Madness Explained: Psychosis and
Human Nature* (Penguin, 2002).

34   **psychological and emotional
adaptation has been far more
difficult:** Willem Rasing, *Too Many
People*; Michael Kral, *The Return
of the Sun: Suicide and Reclamation
Among Inuit of Arctic Canada*
(Oxford University Press, 2019).

34   **a trading post in what is now
Nunavut:** Jean Briggs, "Emotions
Have Many Faces: Inuit Lessons,"

148   *Anthropologica* XLII (2000): 157–164.

35 **"where they hit their children, let babies cry, kiss grown-ups, and make pets of dogs and cats":** Jean Briggs, *Never in Anger*, 74.

36 **joking questions from parents and other adults that must have been confusing and scary to them:** Examples come from Jean Briggs, "In Search of Emotional Meaning," *Ethos* 15 (1987): 8–15, and *Inuit Morality Play* (Yale University Press, 1998).

37 **many of the former residential school children resorted to alcohol:** Piotr Wilk, Alana Maltby, and Martin Cooke, "Residential Schools and the Effects on Indigenous Health and Well-Being in Canada—A Scoping Review," *Public Health Reviews* 38, no. 8 (2017); "What It's Like . . . When Drinking Masks Residential-School Pain," *Globe and Mail*, January 26, 2017, https://www .theglobeandmail.com/life/health -and-fitness/health/what -its-likewhen-drinking-masks -residential-school-pain-health /article33782549/.

38 **we're conditioned not to be a burden to others:** Difficulty handling strong emotions is a strong predictor of suicide. See for example Andrada D. Neacsiu, Caitlin M. Fang, Marcus Rodriguez, and M. Zachary Rosenthal, "Suicidal Behavior and Problems with Emotion Regulation," *Suicide and Life Threatening Behaviors* 48, no. 1 (2018): 52–74.

39 **Data from the coroner's office cited by Jack Hicks indicate that this is not the case:** Jack Hicks, "A Critical Analysis of Myth-Perpetuating Research on Suicide Prevention," *Northern Public Affairs* 6, no. 3 (2018), https://www .researchgate.net/publication /325367875_A_critical_analysis_of _myth-perpetuating_research_on _suicide_prevention.

39 **claimed that the number of teen suicides in the Nunavut town of Kugluktuk fell to zero:** "The Grizzlies: 15 Things About the Groundbreaking New Canadian Film," CBC Radio, April 17, 2019, https://www.cbc.ca/radio/q /blog/the-grizzlies-15-things -about-the-groundbreaking -new-canadian-film-1.5101737; Kugluktuk Grizzlies Lacross, ESPN, 2005. https://www.youtube.com /watch?v=32vBv0-rA0Q; Jack Hicks unpublished data.

39 **multifaceted approaches have been shown to reduce suicides in other communities:** Mary F. Cwik, Lauren Tingey, Alexandra Maschino, Novalene Goklish, Francene Larzelere-Hinton, John Walkup, and Allison Barlow, "Decreases in Suicide Deaths and Attempts Linked to the White Mountain Apache Suicide

Surveillance and Prevention
System, 2001–2012," *American
Journal of Public Health* 106, no. 12
(2016): 2183-2189.

**41 one hundred young Inuit
marched:** "Iqaluit Teens Take to
the Street to Demand More Suicide
Prevention for Nunavummiut,"
CBC News, November 17, 2021.

**41 plans and increased
funding:** Jeff Pelletier, "Nunavut
Suicide Prevention Plan Focuses
on Supporting Young People,"
Nunutsiaq News, October 31,
2024; Tharsha Ravichakaravarthy,
"Nunavut to Spend \$3.3M to Fund
Suicide and Substance Abuse
Prevention Programs," CBC News,
January 10, 2025.

CHAPTER 2
**42 thousands of tiny tropical
islands lush with coconut and
breadfruit trees:** Francis X. Hezel,
Making Sense of Micronesia.

**43 As a person without family
or taro gardens, Lutz was seen as
having special needs:** Catherine
Lutz, *Unnatural Emotions: Everyday
Sentiments on a Micronesian Atoll
and Their Challenge to Western
Theory* (University of Chicago
Press, 1988), 45.

**43 they had no sense of self
inside, distinct from the public
one:** Catherine Lutz, *Unnatural
Emotions*, 96.

43 **"sometimes she seems**   149
to have no soul of her own":
Francis X. Hezel, *Making Sense of
Micronesia*, 25.

**44 what may be the most
ambitious economic and
social development program
ever attempted:** David Boyer,
"Micronesia: The Americanization
of Eden," *National Geographic*, 1967.

**45 sons and daughters of
fishermen had become office and
construction workers:** P. F. Kluge,
*The Edge of Paradise: America in
Micronesia* (Random House, 1991).

**45 whether accepting American
foreign aid had meant selling their
souls:** Mac Marshall, *Weekend
Warriors: Alcohol in a Micronesian
Culture* (Mayfield Publishing
Company, 1979), 34, 116.

**45 most heartbreaking aspect
of this social catastrophe was the
suicide rate:** Donald H. Rubinstein,
"Epidemic Suicide Among
Micronesian Adolescents," *Social
Science & Medicine* 17, no. 10 (1983):
657–665, https://doi.org/10.1016
/0277-9536(83)90372-6.

**46 "and then something seems
to close down on them":** David
Nevin, *The American Touch in
Micronesia* (Norton, 1977), 30.

**46 few suffered from mental
illnesses of any kind:** Francis X.
Hezel, "Micronesia's Hanging
Spree," *Micronesian Independent*,

150   December 31, 1976. See also
"Tragic End for Troubled Youth,"
Micronesian Reporter 14, no. 4
(1976): 8–13; "Suicide Beckons
Micronesia," *Pacific Daily News*,
February 13, 1977; "Suicide
Epidemic Among Micronesian
Youth," *South Pacific Bulletin* 27,
no. 2 (1977): 5–10.

47   **"Much love from Sima":**
Donald H. Rubinstein, "Love and
Suffering: Adolescent Socialization
and Suicide in Micronesia,"
Contemporary Pacific 7, no. 1 (1995):
21–53.

48   **psychologist Stanley Hall
produced the first comprehensive
account:** Stanley Hall, *Adolescence:
Its Psychology and Its Relations
to Physiology, Anthropology,
Sociology, Sex, Crime, and Religion*
(D. Appleton and Company, 1904).

49   **but most did so in trauma-
free ways:** Paul Bohannan, ed.,
African Homicide and Suicide
(Princeton University Press,
1960); Margaret Mead, *Coming of
Age in Samoa* (William Morrow,
1928); Alice Schlegel and Herbert
Barry III, *Adolescence: An
Anthropological Inquiry* (Free Press,
1991); Ruth Benedict, *Patterns of
Culture* (Routledge, 1935).

49   **in more than 180 other
communities around the world:**
Alice Schlegel and Herbert
Barry III, *Adolescence: An
Anthropological Inquiry*.

50   **played a constructive role:**
Thomas Gladwin, *Truk: Man in
Paradise* (Wenner Gren Foundation
for Anthropological Research,
1953).

50   **to bring a relationship back
into alignment by signaling:** D. H.
Rubinstein, "Self-Righteous Anger,
Soft Talk, and Amwúnúmwún
Suicides of Young Men: The
Ambivalent Ethos of Gentleness
and Violence in Truk," paper
presented at the American
Anthropological Association
meetings in Denver, November
15–18, 1984.

50   **now, exact repayment was
expected:** Barbara Demory, *An
Illusion of Surplus: The Effect
of Status Rivalry Upon Family
Food Consumption* (PhD thesis,
University of California, Berkeley,
1976).

51   **growing numbers of children
in this new patriarchy began to
succumb to malnutrition:** Barbara
Demory, *An Illusion of Surplus*.

52   **now fork over some $85
billion annually on children's
allowances:** Richard Laycock,
"Finder Study Reports That Kids
Are Receiving a Collective $85
Billion a Year in Pocket Money,"
Finder.com, December 18, 2023,
https://www.finder.com/kids
-banking/chores-allowance-us
-statistics; Viviana Zelizer, *Pricing
the Priceless Child* (Princeton
University Press, 1985).

52   there was no way for a young Micronesian to explain this: Francis X. Hezel, *Making Sense of Micronesia*, 114; Catherine Lutz, *Unnatural Emotions*, 104.

52   would fill the night air with war cries: Mac Marshall, *Weekend Warriors*, 70.

53   walked over to him, like an actor breaking character: Mac Marshall, *Weekend Warriors*, 113.

53   "It's the quiet ones we lose": *Suicide in Micronesia: Finding a Better Way Out*. A video produced by the Micronesian Seminar, 2004.

54   likened societies to bodies and cultural practices to organs: Bronisław Malinowski, *A Scientific Theory of Culture* (University of North Carolina Press, 1944).

54   "We develop the capacity to feel true awe in church": Clifford Geertz, "The Impact of the Concept of Culture on the Concept of Man," in *Man in Adaptation* (Routledge, 1974).

CHAPTER 3
56   wondering whether he'd made a terrible mistake: Tony Wood, *Russia Without Putin: Money, Power and the Myths of the New Cold War* (Verso, 2018); David Remnick, *Resurrection: The Struggle for a New Russia* (Vintage, 1998).

56   tons of fish rotted onshore while officials in Moscow tried to figure out what to do with them: David Remnick, *Lenin's Tomb: The Last Days of the Soviet Empire* (Vintage, 1994).

00   the leading cause of house fires in the country: *Traumazone*, a film by Adam Curtis, BBC Television, 2022.

57   ruble collapsed and the economy shrank at one point: David Stuckler and Sanjay Basu, "The Post-Communist Mortality Crisis," chapter 2 in *The Body Economic: Why Austerity Kills* (Basic books, 2013).

57   poor people survived on potato peelings: David Stuckler and Sanjay Basu, "The Post-Communist Mortality Crisis."

57   chopped down trees in city parks for firewood: *Traumazone*.

57   Hit men murdered journalists, legislators, and bankers: "Godfather of the Kremlin?" *Forbes*, December 30, 1996 (updated June 6, 2013), https://www.forbes.com /forbes/1996/1230/5815090a .html?sh=728cd41d7562.

57   sometimes had to pursue criminals by bus: Stephen Handelman, "The Russian 'Mafiya,'" *Foreign Affairs*, March 1, 1994.

58   old people rummaging through garbage cans: Boris Yeltsin, *The Struggle for Russia* (Crown, 1994), 272.

152

58   **he realized he'd never faced a problem like this:** Boris Yeltsin, *The Struggle for Russia*, 220.

58   **locked the door, lay down on his back, and closed his eyes:** Boris Yeltsin, *The Struggle for Russia*.

58   **a bodyguard managed to open the door and convinced him to come out:** Boris Yeltsin, *The Struggle for Russia*, 194.

58   **armies of babushkas to march on the main TV station waving photographs of Stalin:** Boris Yeltsin, *The Struggle for Russia*.

58   **would not have fired even if his aides had failed:** Timothy Colton, *Boris Yeltsin: A Life* (Basic Books, 2011).

59   **male life expectancy fell by six years:** David A. Leon et al., "Huge Variation in Russian Mortality Rates 1984–94: Artefact, Alcohol, or What?"

59   **Suicides doubled among middle-aged men:** Elizabeth Brainerd and David M. Cutler, "Autopsy on an Empire: Understanding Mortality in Russia and the Former Soviet Union," *Journal of Economic Perspectives*, 19, no. 1 (2005): 107–130.

59   **can shut it down completely:** Lauri Holmström, Janna Kauppila, Juha Vähätalo, Heiki Huikkuri, and Juhani Junttila, "Sudden Cardiac Death After Alcohol Intake: Classification and Autopsy

Findings," *Scientific Reports* 12, 16771 (2022); Leon Greenberg, "Alcohol in the Body," *Scientific American*, 189, no. 6 (December 1953): 86–91.

59   **lacked signs of blocked arteries or plaque:** David A. Leon, Vladimir M. Shkolnikov, Martin McKee, Nikolay Kiryanov, and Evgueny Andreev, "Alcohol Increases Circulatory Disease Mortality in Russia: Acute and Chronic Effects or Misattribution of Cause?" *International Journal of Epidemiology* 39, no. 5 (2010): 1279–1290.

59   **alcoholism is a huge risk factor for suicide:** Nahid Darvishi, Mehran Farhadi, Tahereh Haghtalab, and Jalal Poorolajal, "Alcohol-Related Risk of Suicidal Ideation, Suicide Attempt, and Completed Suicide: A Meta-Analysis," *PLoS ONE* 10, no. 5 (2015): e0126870; George E. Murphy and Richard D. Wetzel, "The Lifetime Risk of Suicide in Alcoholism," *Archives of General Psychiatry* 47, no. 4, (1990): 383–392, https://psycnet.apa.org/doi/10.1001/archpsyc.1990.01810160083012; William Alex Pridemore and Mitchell B. Chamlin, "A Time-Series Analysis of the Impact of Heavy Drinking on Homicide and Suicide Mortality in Russia, 1956–2002," *Addiction* 101, no. 12 (2006): 1719–1729, https://doi.org/10.1111/j.1360-0443.2006.01631.x; Guilherme Borges, Courtney Bagge, Cheryl J. Cherpital,

Kenneth Conner, Ricardo Orozco, and Ingeborg Rossow, "A Meta-Analysis of Acute Alcohol Use and the Risk of Suicide Attempt," *Psychological Medicine* 47, no. 5 (2017), 949–957, https://doi.org/10.1017/S0033291716002841 (this paper found acute alcohol intoxication increased suicide risk nearly sevenfold).

59   severe alcoholics are roughly a hundred times more likely: George E. Murphy, Richard D. Wetzel, Eli Robins, and Larry McEvoy, "Multiple Risk Factors Predict Suicide in Alcoholism," *Archives of General Psychiatry* 49, no. 6 (1992): 459–463, https://doi.org/10.1001/archpsyc.1992.01820060039006.

60   nearly half of all working-age male suicides were heavy alcohol users: William Alex Pridemore and Mitchell B. Chamlin, "A Time-Series Analysis of the Impact of Heavy Drinking on Homicide and Suicide Mortality in Russia, 1956–2002."

60   "I have a home. But I have nothing to do.": Michael Wines, "An Ailing Russia Lives Through a Tough Life That's Getting Shorter," *New York Times*, December 3, 2000, https://www.nytimes.com/2000/12/03/world/an-ailing-russia-lives-a-tough-life-that-s-getting-shorter.html.

60   developed a culture of endurance, passivity, and

resignation: Daniel Rancour-Lafferiere, *The Slave Soul of Russia: Moral Masochism and the Cult of Suffering* (NYU Press, 1995).

61   what looked like freedom to Western observers was experienced by Russians as existential chaos: Michelle Parsons, *Dying Unneeded: The Cultural Context of the Russian Mortality Crisis* (Vanderbilt University Press, 2014). I'm loosely translating the word "Bespredel"—literally "without limits"—to describe the sense of those times.

61   into old patterns of despair and alcohol-induced psychological stasis: This historical sketch is based on Richard Pipes, *Russia Under the Old Regime* (Simon & Schuster, 1974); Masha Gessen, *The Future Is History: How Totalitarianism Reclaimed Russia* (Riverhead, 2017).

61   peasants, monks, and czars as more or less permanently drunk: Stephen White, *Russia Goes Dry: Alcohol, State and Society* (Cambridge University Press, 1995).

61   alcohol rehab centers: Stephen White, *Russia Goes Dry*, 159.

61   in a third of private homes in some areas: Stephen White, *Russia Goes Dry*, 159.

154   61   **people drank not only perfume:** Stephen White, *Russia Goes Dry*, 19.

61   **became known as the "flying restaurant":** Stephen White, *Russia Goes Dry*, 53, 54.

61   **were consuming, on average, a bottle of vodka every two days:** Stephen White, *Russia Goes Dry*, 165.

61   **half the male population were alcoholics:** Stephen White, *Russia Goes Dry*, 166.

62   **"If you tried to stop them, stones and bottles came flying at your windows":** Stephen White, *Russia Goes Dry*, 147.

62   **some ten million men would be prematurely dead:** The capitalism-blamers include epidemiologists Martin McKee, Martin Bobak, David Cutler and Elizabeth Brainerd, and Vladimir Shkolnikov, as well as political scientist David Stuckler and Dr. Sanjay Basu. As far as I know, all partisans for the theory that the Russian mortality crisis resulted from the legacy of Soviet communism are affiliated with organizations that promote free market economic reforms, including the American Enterprise Institute, the *Economist* magazine, and the Upjohn Institute. See David Stuckler and Sanjay Basu, "The Post-Communist Mortality Crisis," for a discussion of how some communism-blamers may have mishandled the mortality data to arrive at their conclusions. See also: David Stuckler, Lawrence King, and Martin McKee, "The Disappearing Health Effects of Rapid Privatisation: A Case of Statistical Obscurantism?" *Social Science & Medicine* 75, no. 1 (2012): 23–31.

62   **crisis only began to subside with the rise of oil prices and job growth:** Mortality in Russia began falling steeply in 2005. See Elizabeth Brainerd, "Mortality in Russia Since the Fall of the Soviet Union," *Comparative Economic Studies* 63, no. 4 (2021): 557–576, https://doi.org/10.1057/s41294 -021-00169-w. Writer Masha Gessen, who is skeptical that mortality fell in the 2000s, points out that the 2010 census was probably manipulated to make the Russian population appear larger than it really was, and therefore, Russian mortality appears lower than it really was. However, mortality rates aren't generally calculated from census data; they are calculated from death certificates and independent surveys. I have seen no evidence that these became less accurate than in the past after 2005.

62   **large cities, rather than in the much poorer countryside:**

Elizabeth Brainerd and David M. Cutler, "Autopsy on an Empire."

62   it had always been an alien system in Russia: Dale Pesmen, *Russia and Soul* (Cornell University Press, 2000).

62   folk healers refused money: Dale Pesmen, *Russia and Soul*.

63   buying commodities somewhere else in order to sell them at a higher price to your own people was profiteering: Dale Pesmen, *Russia and Soul*.

63   suggested that a Russian version of *Sesame Street* include a segment with children selling lemonade on the street: David Smith, "Muppets in Moscow: The Wild Story Behind Sesame Street in Russia," *The Guardian*, October 18, 2022, https://www.theguardian.com/tv-and-radio/2022/oct/18/muppets-in-moscow-sesame-street-russia-book.

64   ordinary Soviets were always giving each other things: Alena Ledeneva, *Russia's Economy of Favours: Blat, Networking and Informal Exchange* (Cambridge University Press, 1998).

64   how this system descended like an "atom bomb": Svetlana Alexievich, *Secondhand Time: The Last of the Soviets* (Random House, 2017), 19.

65   "What is our national idea now, besides salami?": Svetlana Alexievich, *Secondhand Time*, 54.

65   "You [felt] for others. . . . You're broke? Go to Hell!'": Svetlana Alexievich, *Secondhand Time*, 50.

65   "'Kick the weak in the eyes!'": Svetlana Alexievich, *Secondhand Time*, 158.

65   "Wolves! They came after everyone": Svetlana Alexievich, *Secondhand Time*, 36.

65   "The smell of money filled the air": Svetlana Alexievich, *Secondhand Time*, 162.

65   "'Grandma, where do you think you are going?'": Michelle Parsons, *Dying Unneeded*.

65   "a gargantuan theme park of inconvenience": Nancy Ries, *Russian Talk: Culture and Conversation During Perestroika* (Cornell University Press, 1997), 42.

65   phrases "complete ruin" and "total disaster": Nancy Ries, *Russian Talk*, 44.

66   "abandoned in a hostile world": Dale Pesmen, *Russia and Soul*, 71.

66   the feeling that others no longer had a use for them: Michelle Parsons, *Dying Unneeded*.

156

66   "They still haven't recovered": Svetlana Alexievich, *Secondhand Time*, 162.

66   with the old sharing economy went the whole idea of friendship: Svetlana Alexievich, *Secondhand Time*, 158.

66   "Before, it had seemed like we didn't need money at all": Svetlana Alexievich, *Secondhand Time*, 155.

67   Some of those who took their own lives had fought in World War II: Svetlana Alexievich, *Secondhand Time*, 194.

67   only to set himself on fire in his back garden: Svetlana Alexievich, *Secondhand Time*, 78.

68   "It's like they never had a life of their own": Masha Gessen, "Svetlana Alexievich's Nobel Win," *New Yorker*, October 8, 2015.

68   saw himself as Russia's first truly human head of state: Boris Yeltsin, *The Struggle for Russia*.

68   by virtue of the providential mystique of the classless utopian future: Boris Yeltsin, *The Struggle for Russia*, 193, 196, 288.

69   he seemed to feel their pain, as if he were one of them: Timothy Colton, *Boris Yeltsin: A Life*.

69   "the half-starving, almost ascetic barracks existence": Boris Yeltsin, *The Struggle for Russia*, 62.

70   he'd seen his father arrested and sent to one of Stalin's gulags: Boris Yeltsin, *The Struggle for Russia*, 196.

70   another containing two bottles of vodka and a jar of pickled cucumbers: Boris Yeltsin, *Midnight Diaries* (Public Affairs), 2000.

71   led the musicians in a tipsy rendition of the Russian folk song "Kalinka": Matthew Weaver, "Boris Yeltsin's Magic Moments," *The Guardian*, April 23, 2007, https://www.theguardian.com/news/blog/2007/apr/23/borisyeltsins.

71   you'd have to consume about twenty-five shots of vodka: "How Much Alcohol Can Kill You? It Depends," Healthline, accessed December 9, 2024, https://www.healthline.com/health/alcohol/how-much-alcohol-can-kill-you#number-of-drinks.

71   the better they said they felt—even as their drinking was killing them: Discussed in Michelle Parsons, *Dying Unneeded*.

72   enabling friends to part with things that seemed to come from nowhere: Dale Pesmen, *Russia and Soul*, 188.

72   time spent drinking with friends doesn't count toward your lifespan: Svetlana Alexievich, *Secondhand Time*, 236.

72   **most Russians were fed up with their country's economic experiments:** Masha Gessen, *The Future Is History*, 202.

73   **"No values are left except for the power of the purse":** Svetlana Alexievich, *Secondhand Time*, 270.

73   **"Obedience and love for one's leader":** Masha Gessen, *The Future Is History*, 236.

CHAPTER 4

00   **What he would not otherwise have been able to detect otherwise was how lonely:** Vivek Murthy, *Our Epidemic of Loneliness and Isolation: The U.S. Surgeon General's Advisory on the Healing Effects of Social Connection and Community*, 2023.

74   **halved since 1990:** Daniel Cox, "The State of American Friendship: Change, Challenges, and Loss Findings from the May 2021 American Perspectives Survey," *AEI*, June 8, 2021.

74   **said they felt lonely most of the time:** Bianca DiJulio, Liz Hamel, Cailey Muñana, and Mollyann Brodie, "Loneliness and Social Isolation in the United States, the United Kingdom, and Japan: An International Survey," Kaiser Family Foundation, August 30, 2018.

75   **spend twenty hours less each month socializing:** Vivek Murthy, *Our Epidemic of Loneliness and Isolation*.

75   **such as speeding through a red light or giving the finger to another driver:** *Join or Die: A Film About Why You Should Join a Club*, directed by Pete Davis and Rebecca Davis, 2023, https://www .joinordiefilm.com/; for more recent data on declining social capital, especially among the workers, see Daniel A. Cox and Sam Pressler, "Disconnected: The Growing Class Divide in American Civic Life: Findings from 2024 American Social Capital Survey," American Enterprise Institute, August 22, 2024, https: //www.american surveycenter.org/research /disconnected-places-and-spaces/.

75   **adolescents and young adults were three to four times more likely to die by suicide than their 1950s counterparts:** Robert Putnam, *Bowling Alone: The Collapse and Revival of American Community* (Simon & Schuster, 1999), 262.

76   **suicide rate for middle-aged people with bachelor's degrees had barely budged:** Anne Case and Angus Deaton, *Deaths of Despair and the Future of Capitalism* (Princeton University Press, 2020), 127.

76   **those places where people seem to be most lonely:** Muxin Zhai, Ruby P. Kishan, and Dean Showalter, "Social Capital and Suicidal Behaviors: Evidence from the United States Counties," *Journal of Behavioral and Experimental*

158   *Economics* 98 (2022); Nathan Daniel, Lucia Smith, and Ichiro Kawachi, "State-Level Social Capital and Suicide Mortality in the 50 U.S. States," *Social Science & Medicine* 120 (2014): 269–277.

76   **TV explains only a small fraction of America's social disconnection:** Robert Putnam, *Bowling Alone.*

76   **may be drawn away from the sustaining relationships they desperately need:** Jonathan Haidt, *The Anxious Generation: How the Great Rewiring of Childhood Is Causing an Epidemic of Mental Illness* (Penguin, 2024); see also "The Relationship Between Bullying and Suicide: What We Know and What It Means for Schools," National Center for Injury Prevention and Control (U.S.). Division of Violence Prevention, April 2014, https:// stacks.cdc.gov/view/cdc/34163; Andrew Solomon, "Has Social Media Fueled a Teen Suicide Crisis?" *New Yorker*, October 2024; Kevin Roose, "Can A.I. Be Blamed for a Teen's Suicide?" *New York Times*, October 23, 2024, https:// www.nytimes.com/2024/10/23 /technology/characterai-lawsuit -teen-suicide.html.

77   **which began in the 1970s, long before social media or even personal computers existed:** Jonathan Haidt, *The Anxious Generation*; Jean Twenge, *iGen: Why Today's Super-Connected Kids Are Growing Up Less Rebellious, More Tolerant, Less Happy— and Completely Unprepared for Adulthood—and What That Means for the Rest of Us* (Atria Books, 2017); see also Maya Massing-Schaffer and Jacqueline Nesi, "Cybervictimization and Suicide Risk in Adolescence: An Integrative Model of Social Media and Suicide Theories," *Adolescent Research Review* 5, no. 1 (2020): 49–65, https://psycnet.apa.org/doi/10 .1007/s40894-019-00116-y.

77   **controversies about the data linking social media to suicide:** Eric Levitz, "What the Evidence Really Says About Social Media's Impact on Teens' Mental Health: Did Smartphones Actually 'Destroy' a Generation?" *Vox*, April 12, 2024, https://www.vox.com /24127431/smartphones-young -kids-children-parenting-social -media-teen-mental-health.

77   **prioritizing the welfare of consumers, investment bankers, and corporate shareholders:** Nicholas Lemann, *Transaction Man: The Rise of the Deal and the Decline of the American Dream* (Farrar, Straus and Giroux, 2019).

79   **more than ninety thousand factories closed:** Dan Kaufman, "How NAFTA Broke American Politics," *New York Times Magazine*, September 3, 2024, https://www .nytimes.com/2024/09/03

/magazine/nafta-tarriffs-economy
-trump-kamala-harris.html.

79   **went from having the
country's second highest median
income in 1969 to having the
second highest poverty rate:** Dan
Kaufman, "How NAFTA Broke
American Politics."

80   **through underselling and
other dubiously legal anti-
competitive tactics:** Dana
Mattioli, *The Everything War:
Amazon's Ruthless Quest to Own the
World and Remake Corporate Power*
(Little Brown, 2024).

83   **study in Japan found that
it raises a worker's suicide risk
fourfold:** Akizumi Tsutsumi,
Kazunori Kayaba, Toshiyuki Ojima,
Shizukiyo Ishikawa, and Norito
Kawakami, "Low Control at Work
and the Risk of Suicide in Japanese
Men: A Prospective Cohort Study,"
Psychotherapy and Psychosomatics
76, no. 3 (2007): 177–185; Melody
Almroth, Tomas Hemmingsson,
Katarina Kjellberg, Alma Sörberg
Wallin, Tomas Andersson,
Amanda van der Westhuizen, and
Daniel Falkstedt, "Job Control,
Job Demands and Job Strain and
Suicidal Behaviour Among Three
Million Workers in Sweden,"
*Occupational and Environmental
Medicine* 79 (2022): 681–689,
https://doi.org/10.1136/oemed
-2022-108268.

84   **American children**   159
**experience more changes in
stepfathers, stepmothers, and
residences:** Andrew Cherlin,
*Labor's Love Lost: The Rise and Fall of
the Working-Class Family in America*
(Russell Sage Foundation Books,
2014).

84   **perpetuating an
intergenerational cycle of
thwarted potential:** Angelika H.
Claussen, Joseph R. Holbrook,
Helena J. Hutchins et al., "All in
the Family? A Systematic Review
and Meta-Analysis of Parenting
and Family Environment as Risk
Factors for Attention-Deficit/
Hyperactivity Disorder (ADHD)
in Children," *Prevention Science* 25,
suppl 2 (2024): 249–271, https://
doi.org/10.1007/s11121-022
-01358-4; Shannon E. Cavanagh and
Paula Fomby, "Family Instability,
School Context, and the Academic
Careers of Adolescents," *Sociology
of Education* 85, no. 1 (2012), 81–97,
https://doi.org/10.1177
/0038040711427312.

85   **who doesn't earn enough
for groceries:** Andrew Ross
Sorkin, "Dear C.E.O.: Before
You Give to Charity, Look at
Your Own Workplace," *New York
Times*, December 24, 2019; "From
Paycheck to Pantry: Hunger
in Working America," Oxfam,
November 18, 2014, https://www
.oxfamamerica.org/explore
/research-publications/from

160   -paycheck-to-pantry-hunger
-in-working-america/.

85   **Around 30 percent of
homeless adults have jobs:**
Maureen Sarver, "Why Is It So
Hard for People Experiencing
Homelessness to 'Just Go Get
a Job?'" The Urban Institute,
November 3, 2023; Shannon Vavra
and Steve LeVine, "The Working
Homeless Isn't Just a Tech Bubble
Problem," *Axios*, December 13,
2017.

85   **When workers are made to
feel replaceable and lucky to have
even a lousy job:** Pierre Bourdieu,
"Job Insecurity Is Everywhere
Now," in *Acts of Resistance: Against
the New Myths of Our Time* (Polity,
1998), 81–87; Pierre Bourdieu
(1997) "La précarité est aujourd'hui
partout," paper presented at Lors
des Rencontres européennes contre
la précarité, Grenoble, December
12–13, 1997.

85   **"joy in one's work":** Simone
Weil, *The Need for Roots* (Routledge
2001), 78.

85   **non-BA whites actually
report more pain at age sixty than
at age eighty:** See "The Misery and
Mystery of Pain," chapter 7 of Anne
Case and Angus Deaton, *Deaths of
Despair and the Future of Capitalism*.

85   **were out of the workforce for
health reasons:** Anne Case and
Angus Deaton, *Deaths of Despair
and the Future of Capitalism*, 101.

86   **60 percent of men were either
unemployed or living on disability
payments:** Beth Macy, *Dopesick:
Dealers, Doctors, and the Drug
Company That Addicted America*
(Little Brown, 2018), 125.

86   **amplified the effects of
work injuries, accidents, and the
physical and emotional scars:**
Eric W. de Heer, Marloes M. J. G.
Gerrits, Aartjan T. F. Beekman, Jack
Dekker, Harm W. J. van Marwijk,
Margot W. M. de Waal, et al, "The
Association of Depression and
Anxiety with Pain: A Study from
NESDA," *PLoS ONE* 9, no. 10 (2014):
e106907.

86   **more than doubles the risk of
suicide:** Mark Ilgen, "Pain, Opioids,
and Suicide Mortality in the United
States," *Annals of Internal Medicine*
169 (2018): 498–499.

86   **counties where more people
report chronic pain also tend to
have the highest suicide rates:**
Anne Case and Angus Deaton,
*Deaths of Despair and the Future of
Capitalism*, 126–127.

CHAPTER 5
87   **the suicide rate for military
personnel was lower than that for
same-aged civilians:** Vernon Loeb,
"Military Cites Elevated Rate of
Suicides in Iraq," *Washington Post*,
January 15, 2004; "Suicide Among
Veterans and Other Americans
2001–2014," US Department of
Veterans Affairs, Office of Suicide

Prevention, August 3, 2016 (updated August 2017).

87   **"sandbox wars" had jumped to 124 per 100,000:** Suicides among young male vets who were not linked to the VA health system were lower, but also rose dramatically during this time. See 2019 report on that. The VA's subsequent published reports expanded the age band to eighteen to thirty-four, making simple comparisons difficult. Suicides—for all groups—tend to be higher among people in their early twenties than in their early thirties, so the jump now appeared less marked. Nevertheless, it remained and, as of this writing, little progress on reducing veteran suicide had been made. See Nancy Montgomery, "Study Finds 37 Percent Greater Veteran Suicide Rate Than Reported by VA," *Stars and Stripes*, September 17, 2022, https://www.stripes.com /veterans/2022-09-17/veteran -suicide-rate-study-7363791 .html.

87   **roughly seven times the civilian rate for men in that age group:** In fact, the numbers were even worse. According to a VA study of eight states, twenty-four vets took their lives each day, and another sixteen died from overdoses. Giulia Carbonara, "The Hidden Suicide Epidemic Among U.S. Veterans," *Newsweek*, September 6, 2023.

87   **have been linked to traumatic brain injuries caused by shock waves from heavy artillery:** Dave Phillips, "Pattern of Brain Damage Is Pervasive in Navy SEALs Who Died by Suicide, *New York Times*, June 30, 2024.

87   **those with multiple deployments, only 10 percent:** David Keiran, *Signature Wounds*, 50, 219, 221, 222; see also Michael Schoenbaum, Ronald C. Kessler, Stephen E. Gilman, Lisa J. Colpe, Steven G. Heeringa, Murray B. Stein, Robert J. Ursano, Kenneth Cox, and Army STARRS Collaborators, "Predictors of Suicide and Accident Death in the Army Study to Assess Risk and Resilience in Servicemembers (Army STARRS): Results from the Army Study to Assess Risk and Resilience in Servicemembers (Army STARRS)," *JAMA Psychiatry* 71, no. 5 (2014): 493–503, https://www.ncbi.nlm.nih.gov /pmc/articles/PMC4124912/; "Suicide Among Veterans: Veterans' Issues in Focus," *Rand Health Quarterly* 9, no. 3 (June 30, 2022) 21, https://www.ncbi.nlm.nih .gov/pmc/articles/PMC9242579/.

88   **spark a suicide epidemic on such a scale:** David Kieran, *Signature Wounds: The Untold Story of the Military's Mental Health Crisis* (New York University Press, 2019), 215 ff.

162

88 **Vietnam veterans, contrary to popular belief, have been no more likely to die by suicide than civilians:** Tim A. Bullman, Fatema Z. Akhtar, Sybil W. Morley et al., "Suicide Risk Among US Veterans with Military Service During the Vietnam War," *JAMA Network Open* 6, no. 12 (2023): e2347616, https:// doi.org/10.1001/jamanetworkopen .2023.47616.

88 **among those who had experienced abuse in childhood:** Brandon Nichter, Melanie Hill, Sonya Norman, Moira Haller, and Robert H. Pietrzak, "Associations of Childhood Abuse and Combat Exposure with Suicidal Ideation and Suicide Attempt in U.S. Military Veterans: A Nationally Representative Study," *Journal of Affective Disorders* 276 (2020): 1102–1108, https://doi.org/10.1016 /j.jad.2020.07.120; Keith R. Aronson et al., "The Impact of Adverse Childhood Experiences (ACEs) and Combat Exposure on Mental Health Conditions Among New Post-9/11 Veterans," *Psychological Trauma: Theory, Research, Practice, and Policy* 12, no. 7 (2020): 698, https://doi.org/10 .1037/tra0000614; Nicole R. Morgan et al., "The Interaction of Exposure to Adverse Childhood and Combat Experiences on the Current Mental Health of New Post 9/11 Veterans," *Journal of Community Psychology* 50, no. 1 (2022): 204–220, https://doi.org /10.1002/jcop.22523; Alana Z.

Slavin, Ian C. Fischer, and Robert H. Pietrzak, "Differential Associations of Adverse Childhood Experiences and Mental Health Outcomes in US Military Veterans," *Journal of Psychiatric Research* 172 (2024): 261–265, https://doi.org/10.1016/j .jpsychires.2024.02.040; Robert C. Graziano, Frances M. Aunon, Stefanie T. LoSavio, Eric B. Elbogen, Jean C. Beckham, VA Mid-Atlantic MIRECC Workgroup, Kirsten H. Dillon, "A Network Analysis of Risk Factors for Suicide in Iraq/ Afghanistan-Era Veterans," *Journal of Psychiatric Research* 138 (2021): 264–271, https://doi.org/10.1016/j .jpsychires.2021.03.065.

88 **Child abuse is one of the strongest known risk factors for suicide:** John R. Blosnich, Melissa E. Dichter, Catherine Cerulli, Sonja V. Batten, and Robert M. Bossarte, "Disparities in Adverse Childhood Experiences Among Individuals with a History of Military Service"; see also Maju Mathew Koola, Anthony O. Ahmed, Joseph Sebastian, and Erica J. Duncan, "Childhood Physical and Sexual Abuse Predicts Suicide Risk in a Large Cohort of Veterans," *Primary Care Companion for CNS Disorders* 20, no. 4 (2018): 18m02317, https://doi.org/10.4088 /pcc.18m02317; Sharon Alter, Caroline Wilson, Shengnan Sun, Rachel E. Harris, Zhaoyu Wang, Amanda Vitale, Erin A. Hazlett, Marianne Goodman, Yongchao Ge, Rachel Yehuda, Hanga Galfalvy,

and Fatemeh Haghighi, "The Association of Childhood Trauma with Sleep Disturbances and Risk of Suicide in US Veterans," *Journal of Psychiatric Research* 136 (2021): 54–62.

88 **more severe abuse is associated with greater frequency and seriousness of attempts:** Shanta R. Dube, Robert F. Anda, Vincent J. Felitti , Daniel P. Chapman, David F. Williamson, and Wayne H. Giles, "Childhood Abuse, Household Dysfunction, and the Risk of Attempted Suicide Throughout the Life Span: Findings From the Adverse Childhood Experiences Study," *JAMA* 286, no. 24 (2001): 3089–3096, https:// jamanetwork.com/journals/jama /fullarticle/194504.

88 **four to six times more likely to have experienced sexual or physical abuse than adolescents hospitalized with influenza:** Wilfred Hing-sang Wong, Wen-Hung Kuo, Curt Sobolewski, Inderjeet Bhatia, and Patrick Ip, "The Association Between Child Abuse and Attempted Suicide: A Retrospective Cohort Study," *Crisis: The Journal of Crisis Intervention and Suicide Prevention*, 41, no. 3 (2020): 196–204. https://psycnet.apa.org /fulltext/2019-56088-001.html.

89 **were middle-class kids from rural and suburban towns:** Tim Kane, "Who Bears the Burden? Demographic Characteristics of U.S. Military Recruits Before and After 9/11," The Heritage Foundation, November 7, 2005, https://www.heritage.org/defense /report/who-bears-the-burden -demographic-characteristics-us -military-recruits-and-after-911.

89 **they were twice as likely to have been physically and sexually abused as children:** John R. Blosnich, Melissa E. Dichter, Catherine Cerulli, Sonja V. Batten, and Robert M. Bossarte, "Disparities in Adverse Childhood Experiences Among Individuals with a History of Military Service," *JAMA Psychiatry* 71, no. 9 (2014): 1041–1048, https://doi.org/10.1001 /jamapsychiatry.2014.724. The ACE questionnaire is designed to measure adverse childhood experiences like child abuse and neglect or whether someone grew up with an alcoholic or drug-addicted parent. Previous studies using the ACE questionnaire had found strong correlations between these experiences and adult mental health problems like addiction, depression, and suicide. The ACE questionnaire isn't a perfect instrument. For one thing, it's retrospective. Troubled people tend to see trouble all around them, including in their own pasts. What a mentally healthier person might recall as ordinary family tussles, a depressed person might be more likely to remember as frank domestic violence. Despite this and other caveats, the questionnaire

164   is considered a valid research instrument. See Jochen Hardt and Micheal Rutter, "Validity of Adult Retrospective Reports of Adverse Childhood Experiences: Review of the Evidence," *Journal of Child Psychology and Psychiatry* 45 (2004): 260–273, https://doi.org/10.1111 /j.1469-7610.2004.00218.x; Emily M. Zarse, Mallory R. Neff, Rachel Yoder, Leslie Hulvershorn, Joanna E. Chambers, and R. Andrew Chambers, "The Adverse Childhood Experiences Questionnaire: Two Decades of Research on Childhood Trauma as a Primary Cause of Adult Mental Illness, Addiction, and Medical Diseases," *Cogent Medicine* 6, no. 1 (2019), https://doi.org/1 0.1080/2331205X.2019.1581447; Barnabás Oláh, Zita Fekete, Ildikó Kuritárné Szabó, and Beáta Kovács-Tóth, "Validity and Reliability of the 10-Item Adverse Childhood Experiences Questionnaire (ACE-10) Among Adolescents in the Child Welfare System," *Frontiers in Public Health* 11 (November 2023), https://www.frontiersin.org /journals/public-health/articles /10.3389/fpubh.2023.1258798/full.

89   Australian child sexual abuse survivors were found to be ten to thirteen times more likely to die by suicide: Angela Plunkett, Brian O'Toole, Heather Swanston, R. Kim Oates, Sandra Shrimpton, and Patrick Parkinson, "Suicide Risk Following Child Sexual Abuse," *Ambulatory Pediatrics* 1, no. 5 (2001): 262–266; see also Maju Mathew

Koola, Anthony O. Ahmed, Joseph Sebastian, and Erica J. Duncan, "Childhood Physical and Sexual Abuse Predicts Suicide Risk in a Large Cohort of Veterans"; Sharon Alter, Caroline Wilson, Shengnan Sun, Rachel E. Harris, Zhaoyu Wang, Amanda Vitale, Erin A. Hazlett, Marianne Goodman, Yongchao Ge, Rachel Yehuda, Hanga Galfalvy, and Fatemeh Haghighi, "The Association of Childhood Trauma with Sleep Disturbances and Risk of Suicide in US Veterans," *Journal of Psychiatric Research* 136 (2021): 54–62.

90   moral injury: Brett T. Litz, Nathan Stein, Eileen Delaney, Leslie Lebowitz, William P. Nash, Caroline Silva, and Shira Maguen, "Moral Injury and Moral Repair in War Veterans: A Preliminary Model and Intervention Strategy," *Clinical Psychology Review* 29, no. 8 (December 2009): 695–706.

91   deep loneliness as a result: Eyal Press, "The Wounds of the Drone Warrior," *New York Times Magazine,* June 13, 2018; Dexter Filkins, "Atonement," *New Yorker,* October 22, 2012; Tony Doukoupil, "A New Theory of PTSD and Veterans: Moral Injury," *Newsweek,* December 3, 2012.

92   does not depend on battle experiences: Eyal Press, "The Wounds of the Drone Warrior," *New York Times Magazine,* June 13, 2018.

93   **how preoccupied these men were, in life and in their dreams, not just by battlefield horrors, but also by childhood ones:** W. R. D. Fairbairn, "The Repression and the Return of Bad Objects (With Special Reference to the 'War Neuroses')" (1943), in *Psychoanalytic Studies of the Personality* (Routledge & Kegan Paul, 1952) 59–81.

93   **Pierre Janet:** O. Van der Hart & R. Horst, "The Dissociation Theory of Pierre Janet," *Journal of Traumatic Stress* 2, no. 4 (1989): 397–412.

94   **the hated self remained buried in the basement of the mind like an evil spirit:** W. R. D. Fairbairn, "The War Neuroses; Their Nature and Significance," *British Medical Journal* 1 (1943): 183–186.

94   **Only one of the neuropsychiatric cases:** See J. S. Kasanin, C. Rhode, & E. Wertheimer, "Observations from a Veterans' Clinic on Childhood Factors in Military Adjustment," *American Journal of Orthopsychiatry* 16, no. 4 (1946): 640–659.

95   **is what really causes the psyche to crack:** Sandor Ferenczi, "Confusion of Tongues Between Adults and the Child. The Language of Tenderness and of Passion" (1933), in *Final Contributions to the Problems and Methods of Psycho-Analysis* (Karnac Books, 1980), 156–167. Also see "Confusion of Tongues Between the Adults and the Child (The Language of Tenderness and of Passion)," *International Journal of Psycho-Analysis* 30 (1949): 225–231.

95   **whether she'd like him to find her a new kind of mother, she said no:** Harry Guntrip, "My Experience of Analysis with Fairbairn and Winnicott—(How Complete a Result Does Psycho-Analytic Therapy Achieve?)," *International Review of Psycho-Analysis* 2 (1975): 145–156; David Celani, *The Illusion of Love* (Columbia University Press, 1996).

95   **a war against the self:** Years later, psychiatrist Judith Herman also observed that child-abuse survivors were overwhelmingly likely to blame themselves, rather than their parents. See "Child Abuse," Chapter 5 of *Trauma and Recovery* (Basic Books, 1977).

95   **the battlefields of childhood:** J. S. Kasanin, C. Rhode, and E. Wertheimer, "Observations from a Veterans' Clinic on Childhood Factors in Military Adjustment," *American Journal of Orthopsychiatry* 16, no. 4 (1946): 640–659.

97   **but because he couldn't stand to be in his own skin:** Claude AnShin Thomas, *At Hell's Gate: A Soldier's Journey* (Shambhala, 2004), 40–42.

CHAPTER 6

101 **"the internal world, devious, contradictory, labyrinthine":** Al Alvarez, *The Savage God.*

101 **treatments have helped countless suicidal patients survive:** Stephen Briggs, Gopalakrishnan Netuveli, Nick Gould et al., "The Effectiveness of Psychoanalytic/Psychodynamic Psychotherapy for Reducing Suicide Attempts and Self-Harm: Systematic Review and Meta-Analysis," *British Journal of Psychiatry* 214, no. 6 (2019): 320–328. https://doi.org/10.1192/bjp.2019.33.

101 **talking cures can be very effective:** S. Briggs, G. Netuveli, N. Gould, et al. "The Effectiveness of Psychoanalytic/Psychodynamic Psychotherapy for Reducing Suicide Attempts and Self-Harm: Systematic Review and Meta-Analysis," *British Journal of Psychiatry* 214, no. 6 (2019): 320-328; see also M. Schechter, M. J. Goldblatt, E. Ronningstam, & B. Herbstman, "The Psychoanalytic Study of Suicide, Part I: An Integration of Contemporary Theory and Research," *Journal of the American Psychoanalytic Association* 70, no. 1 (2022): 103–137; M. Schechter, M. J. Goldblatt, E. Ronningstam, & B. Herbstman, "The Psychoanalytic Study of Suicide, Part II: An Integration of Theory, Research, and Clinical Practice," *Journal of the American*

Psychoanalytic Association 70, no. 1 (February 2022): 139–166; and J. G. Tillman. "Disillusionment and Suicidality: When a Developmental Necessity Becomes a Clinical Challenge," *Journal of the American Psychoanalytic Association* 66, no. 2 (2018): 225–242.

102 **suppresses the parts of that same organ:** B. A. Van der Kolk, "The Trauma Spectrum: The Interaction of Biological and Social Events in the Genesis of the Trauma Response," *Journal of Traumatic Stress* 1, no. 3 (1988): 273–290; Pierre Janet, *Psychological Healing: A Historical and Clinical Study* (Martino Fine Books, 2019); Judith Herman, *Trauma and Recovery: The Aftermath of Violence—from Domestic Abuse to Political Terror* (Basic Books, 1997).

103 **makes soapstone carvings of children, giving each one an Arabic name:** Chris J. Antal, Peter D. Yeomans, Rotunda East, Douglas W. Hickey, Solomon Kalkstein, Kimberly M. Brown, and Dana S. Kaminstein, "Transforming Veteran Identity Through Community Engagement: A Chaplain–Psychologist Collaboration to Address Moral Injury," *Journal of Humanistic Psychology* 63, no. 6 (2023): 801–826.

103 **A retired army chaplain and a psychologist led the men:** Edward Tick, *War and the Soul:*

Healing Our Nation's Veterans from Post-Traumatic Stress Disorder (Quest Books, 2005).

104 **and may have served as a form of communal healing:** Girija Kaimal, "How Art Can Heal," *American Scientist* 108, no. 4 (July-August 2020): 228; see also Susan Magsamen and Ivy Ross, *Your Brain on Art* (Random House, 2023).

104 **writing, drama, and art therapy:** Girija Kaimal, Jacqueline P. Jones, Rebekka Dieterich-Hartwell & Xi Wang, "Long-Term Art Therapy Clinical Interventions with Military Service Members with Traumatic Brain Injury and Post-Traumatic Stress: Findings from a Mixed Methods Program Evaluation Study," *Military Psychology* 33, no. 1 (2021): 29–40; Heike Gerger, Christoph Patrick Werner, Jens Gaab, and Pim Cuijpers, "Comparative Efficacy and Acceptability of Expressive Writing Treatments Compared with Psychotherapy, Other Writing Treatments, and Waiting List Control for Adult Trauma Survivors: A Systematic Review and Network Meta-Analysis," *Psychological Medicine* 52, no. 15 (2021), 3484–3496, https://doi .org/10.1017/S0033291721000143.

104 **can reduce PTSD symptoms in veterans and other trauma survivors:** Gemma Wilson-Menzfeld and Jonathan Ackley, "The Theatre as Therapy for Military Veterans? Exploring the Mechanisms Which Impact Psychosocial Well-Being and Social Connections During Theatre-Based Programmes," *Arts and Health* 15, no. 1 (2023): 53–70; see also Bessel van der Kolk, *The Body Keeps the Score*, chapter 20; Alisha Ali, Stephan Wolfert, and Bruce D. Homer, "In the Service of Science: Veteran-Led Research in the Investigation of a Theatre-Based Posttraumatic Stress Disorder Treatment," *Journal of Humanistic Psychology* 63, no. 6 (2023): 782–800, https://doi.org/10.1177 /0022167819839907.

104 **a pebble that looked like a face:** "South African Cave Pebble Outshines Treasures at British Museum," Reuters, November 26, 2016, https://www.reuters.com /article/world/south-african-cave -pebble-outshines-treasures -at-british-museum-idUSK BN13L0FT/. See also Anjan Chaterjee, *The Aesthetic Brain: How We Evolved to Desire Beauty and Enjoy Art* (Oxford University Press, 2015).

104 **touches something inside us that philosophers and scientists have been struggling to define:** Anjan Chaterjee, *The Aesthetic Brain.*

105 **the feeling that your feelings are respected:** Jessica Benjamin, *Beyond Doer and Done to: Recognition Theory, Intersubjectivity and the Third* (Routledge, 2017).

168   105   **Spanish poet Federico García Lorca called it** *duende*: Federico García Lorca, "Theory and play of the duende," 1933. Translated by A.S. Kline, 2007, https://www.poetryintranslation .com/PITBR/Spanish/Lorca Duende.php. Thanks to Marc Ribot for alerting me to this.

108   **the effect on the soul of writing such poetry, Alvarez suggests:** Al Alvarez, *The Savage God*, 261.

108   **"terrible, but utterly natural reaction to the strained, narrow, unnatural necessities":** Al Alvarez, *The Savage God*, 284.

108   **genuinely enduring happiness is not possible, it cannot be the subject of art:** Arthur Schopenhauer, *The World as Will and Idea*, volume 1, book 4.

109   **"what it means to want to escape from these things":** T. S. Eliot. "Tradition and the Individual Talent" in *The Sacred Wood: Essays on Poetry and Criticism* (1920).

110   **deliberately accelerated by ignoring his treatment and eating only sporadically:** D. Felisati and G. Sperati, "Famous Figures: Franz Kafka (1883–1924)," *Acta Otorhinolaryngologica Italica* 25, no. 5 (2005): 328–332, https://www .ncbi.nlm.nih.gov/pmc/articles /PMC2639911/.

111   **they can sometimes reduce suicidal thoughts and plans:** Richard J. Zeifman, Nikhita Singhal, Leah Breslow, and Cory R. Weissman, "On the Relationship Between Classic Psychedelics and Suicidality: A Systematic Review," *ACS Pharmacology & Translational Science* 4, no. 2 (2021): 436–451.

111   **by helping people see their problems as part of the human condition:** Jennifer M. Mitchell, Marcella Ot'alora, Bessel van der Kolk et al., "MDMA-Assisted Therapy for Moderate to Severe PTSD: A Randomized, Placebo-Controlled Phase 3 Trial," *Nature Medicine* 29 (2023): 2473–2480, https://doi.org/10.1038/s41591 -023-02565-4; Jessica Kelleher Rabon, Jameson K. Hirsch, Andrea R. Kaniuka, Fuschia Sirois, Byron D. Brooks, and Kristin Neff, "Self-Compassion and Suicide Risk in Veterans: When the Going Gets Tough, Do the Tough Benefit More from Self-Compassion?" *Mindfulness* 10 (2019): 2544–2554, https://psycnet.apa.org/doi/10 .1007/s12671-019-01221-8; C. J. Healy, Kellie Ann Lee, and Wendy D'Andrea, "Using Psychedelics with Therapeutic Intent Is Associated with Lower Shame and Complex Trauma Symptoms in Adults with Histories of Child Maltreatment," *Chronic Stress* 5 (2021), https://doi.org/10 .1177/24705470211029881.

111 **claimed psychedelics have the potential to end war and exploitation:** Caty Enders, "How Psychedelic Research Got High on Its Own Supply," *New York Times*, August 23, 2024, https://www .nytimes.com/2024/08/23/opinion /psychedelics-mdma-mental -health.html.

111 **for some troubled people, the drugs seem to help:** Richard J. Zeifman, Nikhita Singhal, Rafael G. Dos Santos, Rafael F. Sanches, Flávia de Lima Osório, Jaime E. C. Hallak, and Cory R. Weissman, "Rapid and Sustained Decreases in Suicidality Following a Single Dose of Ayahuasca Among Individuals with Recurrent Major Depressive Disorder: Results from an Open-Label Trial," *Psychopharmacology (Berl)* 238, no. 2 (2021): 453–459; Richard J. Zeifman, Dengdeng Yu, Nikhita Singhal, Guan Wang, Sandeep M. Nayak, and Cory R. Weissman, "Decreases in Suicidality Following Psychedelic Therapy: A Meta-Analysis of Individual Patient Data Across Clinical Trials," *Journal of Clinical Psychiatry* 83, no. 2 (2022): 21r14057, https://doi.org/10.4088 /jcp.21r14057.

111 **MRI studies suggest psychedelics make the brain less modular:** Robin L. Carhart-Harris, "The Entropic Brain—Revisited," *Neuropharmacology* 142 (2018): 167–178.

112 **which have also helped some suicidal people:** Cecilia Njenga, Parashar Pravin Ramanuj, Frederico Jose Coelho de Magalhaes, and Harold Alan Pincus, "New and Emerging Treatments for Major Depressive Disorder," *British Medical Journal* 386, no. 8 (2024): e073823, https://doi.org/10.1136 /bmj-2022-073823.

112 **enabling a more creative, less rigid sense of self:** Rosalind Watts, Camilla Day, Jacob Krzanowski, David Nutt, and Robin Carhart-Harris, "Patients' Accounts of Increased 'Connectedness' and 'Acceptance' After Psilocybin for Treatment-Resistant Depression," *Journal of Humanistic Psychology* 57, no. 5 (2017): 520–564, https://doi .org/10.1177/0022167817709585.

112 **rather than as uniquely personal and shameful defects:** Jennifer M. Mitchell, Marcella Ot'alora, Bessel van der Kolk et al., "MDMA-Assisted Therapy for Moderate to Severe PTSD."

112 **also seem to increase brain levels of oxytocin:** Romain Nardou, Edward Sawyer, Young Jun Song et al., "Psychedelics Reopen the Social Reward Learning Critical Period," *Nature* 618 (2023): 790–798.

112 **real changes in their lives:** R. Watts, C. Day, J. Krzanowski, D. Nutt, and R. Carhart-Harris, "Patients' Accounts of Increased 'Connectedness' and 'Acceptance' After Psilocybin for

170   Treatment-Resistant Depression,"
Journal of Humanistic Psychology 57,
no. 5 (2017): 520–564.

**113   effects of psychedelics fade
after a few months or years:** See
for example, Rafael G. dos Santos,
Rafael Faria Sanches, and Flávia de
Lima Osório, "Long-Term Effects
of Ayahuasca in Patients with
Recurrent Depression: A 5-Year
Qualitative Follow-Up," *Archives of
Clinical Psychiatry* 45, no. 1 (2018):
22–24, http://dx.doi.org/10.1590
/0101-60830000000149.

CONCLUSION
115   most suicidogenic of all:
Brett Pelham et al., "A Truly
Global, Non-WEIRD Examination
of Collectivism: The Global
Collectivism Index (GCI)," *Current
Research in Ecological and Social
Psychology* 3 (2022): 100030; M.
Eskin et al., "Is Individualism
Suicidogenic? Findings from a
Multinational Study of Young
Adults from 12 Countries," *Front
Psychiatry* 11 (April 3, 2020): 259.
This paper found an inconsistent
association between country-level
individualism and suicide, but
this could be because it's the shift
from collectivism to individualism
that causes the problem. Societies
that have been individualistic for
many generations, such as those
of Western Europe, may have
developed cultural, social, and
economic coping mechanisms,
including a strong welfare state and

a demonstrative love culture. This
is consistent with the findings of
this study: M. Lenzi, E. Colucci,
and H. Minas. "Suicide, Culture,
and Society from a Cross-National
Perspective," *Cross-Cultural
Research* 46, no. 1 (2011): 50–71,
https://doi.org/10.1177/1069
397111424036 (original work
published 2012).

**115   among farmers in the
US:** Debbie Weingarten, "Why
Are America's Farmers Killing
Themselves?" *The Guardian*,
December 11, 2018.

115   South America: Charlotte
Shaw, Jaimee Stuart, Troy Thomas,
and Kairi Kõlves, "Suicidal
Behaviour and Ideation in Guyana:
A Systematic Literature Review,"
Lancet Regional Health-Americas 11
(2022): 100253, https://doi.org/10
.1016/j.lana.2022.100253.

115   and India: Nanda Kishore
Kannuri and Sushrut Jadhav,
"Cultivating Distress: Cotton,
Caste and Farmer Suicides in India,"
Anthropology & Medicine 28, no. 4
(2021): 558–575, https://doi.org/10
.1080/13648470.2021.1993630.

116   Irish Travellers: Mary
Rose Walker, "Suicide and Irish
Travellers," in *Making Sense of
Suicide?* (Brill, 2011).

**118   He and Durkheim knew of
each other's work, but disagreed:**
Joan Aldous, Émile Durkheim, and
Ferdinand Tönnies, "An Exchange

Between Durkheim and Tönnies on the Nature of Social Relations, with an Introduction by Joan Aldous," *American Journal of Sociology* 77, no. 6 (1972).

118 **mental health suffers when societies come to place greater emphasis on material goods than on relationships:** See also Johann Hari, *Lost Connections: Uncovering the Real Causes of Depression and the Unexpected Solutions* (Bloomsbury, 2018).

118 **traces a series of market transitions in societies around the world:** David Graeber, *Debt: The First 5,000 Years* (Melville House, 2012).

118 **roughly corresponding to Tönnies:** David Luban, "Indebted," *Dissent* 59, no. 2 (Spring 2012): 102–106, https://muse.jhu.edu /article/469415.

119 **The suicide rate has also risen sharply:** Mark Mohan Kaggwa, Godfrey Zari Rukundo, Edith K Wakida, Samuel Maling, Baker Makaya Sserumaga, Letizia Maria Atim, and Celestino Obua, "Suicide and Suicide Attempts Among Patients Attending Primary Health Care Facilities in Uganda: A Medical Records Review, Risk Management and Healthcare Policy," *Risk Management and Healthcare Policy* 15 (2022): 703–711, https://doi.org/10.2147/RMHP. S358187; Dorothy Kizza, Heidi Hjelmeland, Eugene Kinyanda,

and Birthe Loa Knizek, "Alcohol and Suicide in Postconflict Northern Uganda. A Qualitative Psychological Autopsy Study," *Crisis* 33, no 2 (2012), https://doi .org/10.1027/0227-5910/a000119; Dorothy Kizza, Birthe Loa Knizek, Eugene Kinyanda, and Heidi Hjelmeland, "Men in Despair: A Qualitative Psychological Autopsy Study of Suicide in Northern Uganda," *Transcultural Psychiatry* 49, no. 5 (2012): 696–717, https:// doi.org/10.1177/1363461512459490.

120 **the sometimes-fragile ties of family and friendship:** Charles Taylor, *Sources of the Self: The Making of Modern Identity* (Harvard University Press, 1992).

120 **"The fact of thought became itself an object of thought":** Karl Jaspers, "The Axial Age of Human History: A Base for the Unity of Mankind," *Commentary*, November 1948.

122 **furthered economic change:** Taylor, *Sources of the Self*, 206.

122 **elaborate on Smith's ideas in a series of pamphlets and magazine essays:** Robert Dorfman, "Thomas Robert Malthus and David Ricardo," *Journal of Economic Perspectives* 3, no. 3 (Summer 1989): 153–164.

123 **pushed many, if not most, workers into meaningless, alienating jobs at subsistence wages:** Karl Marx, *Economic and*

172 *Philosophic Manuscripts of 1844*, trans. Martin Milligan (Moscow: Progress Publishers, 1959).

124 **"but that he was now existing under the physical conditions that denied the human shape of life":** Karl Polanyi, *The Great Transformation: The Political and Economic Origins of Our Time* (1944) (Beacon Press, 2001), Kindle edition, 2785.

124 **the degradation of his natural environment and his relationship to it:** Karl Polanyi, *The Great Transformation*, Kindle edition, 3400.

124 **"crude, callous beings":** Karl Polanyi, *The Great Transformation*, Kindle edition, 3389.

124 **were dying out, even where there had been no violence involved in their conquest:** Margaret Mead, *The Changing Culture of an Indian Tribe*, WHR Rivers Essays on the Depopulation of Melanesia, 1922, reprint edition (Cambridge University Press, 2015).

125 **Commerce, it was hoped, would be "civilizing":** See, for example, Thomas Friedman, "Foreign Affairs Big Mac I," *New York Times*, December 8, 1996.

127 **who ordered them to strive for the glorious communist future, not to live for themselves:** Masha Gessen, *The Future Is History*.

127 **trauma tends to shut down the very parts of the brain that help us organize and express our thoughts:** Bessel van der Kolk, *The Body Keeps the Score*.

129 **because of the erosion of the checks and balances that were supposed to be built into political liberalism:** Robert Kuttner, "Blaming Liberalism," *New York Review of Books*, November 21, 2019.

129 **held conferences on declining social capital:** William J. Clinton, "Remarks at the Third Session of the White House Conference on the New Economy," The American Presidency Project, April 5, 2000, https://www.presidency.ucsb.edu/documents/remarks-the-third-session-the-white-house-conference-the-new-economy; Robert McFadden, "Amitai Etzioni, 94, Dies; Envisioned a Society Built on the Common Good," *New York Times*, June 1, 2023.

130 **"destroys human roots":** Quotes in Robert Zaretsky, *The Subversive Simone Weil: A Life in Five Ideas* (University of Chicago Press, 2001).

130 **"The world was divided up differently":** Svetlana Alexievich, *Secondhand Time*.

132 **We are kinder to one another when we don't feel threatened:** See also Arjun Jayadev and Robert Johnson, *Tides and Prejudice: Racial*

Attitudes During Downturns in the United States, 1979–2014. Referred to in Arlie Russell Hochschild, *Stolen Pride: Loss, Shame, and the Rise of the Right* (The New Press, 2024).

133   **"a sad portrait of the pure egoist":** Steven Lukes, *Emile Durkheim, His Life and Work: A Historical and Critical Study* (Stanford University Press, 1985), 80.

Columbia Global Reports is a nonprofit publishing imprint from Columbia University that commissions authors to produce works of original thinking and on-site reporting from all over the world, on a wide range of topics. Our books are short—novella-length, and readable in a few hours—but ambitious. They offer new ways of looking at and understanding the major issues of our time. Most readers are curious and busy. Our books are for them.

If this book changed the way you look at the world, and if you would like to support our mission, consider making a gift to Columbia Global Reports to help us share new ideas and stories.

Visit globalreports.columbia.edu to support our upcoming books, subscribe to our newsletter, and learn more about Columbia Global Reports. Thank you for being part of our community of readers and supporters.